*The Young
Person's Guide to*

HEALTH
AND
WELLNESS

"*The Young Person's Guide to Health and Wellness* is for smart, ambitious teenagers who want to live up to their physical, intellectual, and psychological potential—now and into the future. Those of us past our formative years will wish we'd had it (its mind/body approach is astute and perfectly integrated)! Its advice is designed to stay with readers, even as they grow and adapt to new challenges. It's practical, candid, and unflinching, addressing real-life topics that gauzier books just ignore. Readers will feel that the *Guide* is talking to them, anticipating their concerns, helping them to act responsibly towards themselves and in the world. I have never seen topics as varied as nutrition, empathy, STDs, and choice-making discussed so effectively in one compact volume. Teenagers, as well as their teachers, parents, and health-care providers, should read this book."

—Heather Berlin, PhD, Mount Sinai Health System

"Dr. Friedberg's *Young Person's Guide* offers so much sane, sound advice that it should be a primary reference for any teenager navigating their life's journey. I will enthusiastically recommend it to all my younger patients. In particular, I like the *Guide*'s emphasis on developing good habits that last a lifetime, since (as I tell all my patients) staying well is just as important as getting well."

—Albert Levy, MD, Director, Manhattan Family Practice

"*The Young Person's Guide* is full of practical wisdom, showing young people how to set their sails towards optimal physical, mental, and emotional well-being. It will help them take stock of their current health and wellness, and design a strategy to work on each domain of wellness over time. Its approach is nonjudgmental, and it reminds readers that they don't need to tackle every domain of health and wellness at once. Rather, it helps readers identify those areas to focus on right now. From good nutrition to healthy habits, from self-reflection to building sound relationships, the *Guide* encapsulates much of what I practice in my own life, and offer my patients in my Integrative Medicine practice."

—Zachary Mulvihill, MD, Integrative Medicine, Weill Cornell Medicine

"As an educator and a parent, I am confident that this *Guide* will not only engage readers, but become a lasting part of their journey to health and wellness. Its accessible and practical approach encourages readers to explore key areas such as healthy eating, building meaningful relationships, and fostering a sense of community. The ten tenets, at the heart of this book, serve as a roadmap for young people to set goals, improve their physical and emotional well-being, and navigate the challenges of making lasting change. As they face obstacles, this *Guide* will be a trusted resource they can return to time and again to lead healthier and more fulfilling lives."

—Simon Owen-Williams, educational leader

The Young Person's Guide to

HEALTH AND WELLNESS

Keep Fit, Think Smart, Get the Most from Your Life

Ahron Friedberg, MD
with Sandra Sherman, JD, PhD

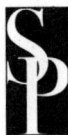

Skyhorse Publishing

Skyhorse Publishing books may be purchased in bulk at special discounts for sales promotion, corporate gifts, fund-raising, or educational purposes. Special editions can also be created to specifications. For details, contact the Special Sales Department, Skyhorse Publishing, 307 West 36th Street, 11th Floor, New York, NY 10018 or info@skyhorsepublishing.com.

Skyhorse® and Skyhorse Publishing® are registered trademarks of Skyhorse Publishing, Inc.®, a Delaware corporation.

Visit our website at www.skyhorsepublishing.com.

Please follow our publisher Tony Lyons on Instagram @tonylyonsisuncertain.

10 9 8 7 6 5 4 3 2 1

Library of Congress Cataloging-in-Publication Data is available on file.

Cover design by David Ter-Avanesyan

Print ISBN: 978-1-5107-8456-7
Ebook ISBN: 978-1-5107-8457-4

Printed in the United States of America

To my children
Sarah, Jacob, and Raquel

Contents

Acknowledgments

I'd like to acknowledge the various institutions and people that made this *Guide* possible. Several local schools in New York City and the surrounding area have referred bright young people to me to work with over the years. These include Horace Mann, Riverdale, Dalton, Trinity, and PS 6, as well as schools in the Great Neck area of Long Island where I live. I also want to thank members of the Portledge Committee on Health and Wellness, where these principles were discussed and vetted. A special thanks to Simon Owen-Williams, head of school at Portledge, for his expertise, encouragement, and support in undertaking this *Guide*. Finally, my deep appreciation to Dr. Sandra Sherman for her tireless efforts in putting our shared vision into elegant prose.

Foreword

I'm a child and adolescent psychiatrist, as well as a father of six. I think about young people a lot. I listen to their problems, share their challenges, and help them develop strategies to become their best selves. But I still wonder how I can ensure that a young person will develop the commitment to remain on track. How can I encourage them to keep thinking about where they're going, what they're doing, and how it will turn out if they choose one path over another? No psychiatrist—or parent, teacher, or friend—can offer all the support a young person needs, whether they're facing everyday issues or real crises. No one can anticipate all the concerns that arise in a young person's life, let alone be there all the time with immediate support. Sometimes, I just hold my breath and hope.

But after reading *The Young Person's Guide to Health and Wellness*, I won't hold my breath quite so often, and my expressions of hope will feel more grounded. This is a terrific book, which young people can turn to again and again. It will be useful no matter where they find themselves. It displays a type of multidimensional understanding that is at once practical, emotionally aware, and reassuring. Most importantly, its advice is never simplistic ("Do this, do that"). Instead, it makes a virtue of nuance. It helps young people adapt its principles to their individual, endlessly changing needs. This is what it *should* do, because unless young people actively—attentively!—participate in designing their own futures, they won't remain engaged in that effort over the long haul. The *Guide* is about the work that's required to *continue* making good choices, even as life presents new, often unexpected challenges.

I use the term "work" because the *Guide* offers an antidote to passivity, the "whatever" shrug that leaves the future to chance. Dr. Friedberg demonstrates that young people have more control over their lives than they think they do, so long as they make good choices and follow through—that is, so long as they keep on working to become their best selves. The *Guide* offers real-world advice on how to make good choices, and then deploy those choices as the basis of good, sustaining habits. The *Guide* is not just about what to do now, but about how to connect "now" with the rest of one's life. It allows young people to envision their lives as an ongoing construction project, rather than just a series of disconnected one-off responses to the grind of daily existence. In this sense, it is hugely encouraging, even as it makes clear that real work is required to make the most of everyday challenges. It elevates the importance of *now* as integral to a perspective based on *years-from-now*.

The idea of integrating the immediate and the long term might be termed "holistic," an approach that requires us to weigh the consequences of acting before we act. In effect, we act based on the *course* of our lives. Thus, while we inhabit the moment, we understand its connection to what's next. And next after that. It's the best way to ensure stability in our lives, as well as the success of our plans. Yet, because many young people don't know how to act holistically—or think that doing so will make life less fun—Dr. Friedberg shows them how, while still finding joy every day. He demonstrates, for example, the importance of slowing down; making cost/benefit analyses; calculating the effect of our actions on people around us. He explains how to switch gears when we sense that something isn't working, so that we don't continue down some unrewarding path. Always, he emphasizes cultivating consciousness over indifference, passivity, or the sense that things will work out . . . somehow. In the universe of the *Guide*, "somehow" is not an option.

Of course, this is a book for thoughtful young people. But if a young person isn't naturally thoughtful, the *Guide* will show them how to practice thoughtfulness, for example by adopting habits like self-reflection, mindfulness, and empathy (thoughtfulness extends to how we interact with others). It will encourage them to *share* what they think with others as a way of deepening their capacity to understand their lives. It will even teach them to read the labels on foods, rather than grab whatever is at eye level. I want to emphasize this last point as one among many ways that the *Guide*—holistically—integrates the physical aspects of life into those that are psychological, intellectual, and emotional. Throughout, the *Guide* demonstrates the importance of the mind-body nexus. Taking care of one's body requires mental effort; conversely, when we suffer physically, our mental stability suffers too. The *Guide* helps young people to maintain their optimal mind-body connectivity.

As Dr. Friedberg explains in the introduction, the *Guide* is organized around ten "tenets," or principles, that help young people approach every day, every problem, holistically. These include tenets such as "Healthy habits strengthen you" and "Nurturing a sound mind is important to physical health." In discussing each tenet, Dr. Friedberg provides immediately useful, practical advice that meets young people where they are, and that they can adapt to their own specific needs. Dr. Friedberg has an uncanny knack for finding the right balance between granting young people leeway and setting boundaries for their own long-term well-being. When he examines sensitive subjects such as gender identity and body image, he is candid, empathetic, and abundantly useful in ways that help young people work through their issues. He helps them to formulate issues so that they can think about them and broach them with friends, family, and professionals. There are no *obiter dicta* here. No piety or sentimentality. Just sound advice. Just strategies for coping and, ultimately, succeeding in terms that each young person defines for themselves.

I keep coming back to self-definition, since it's the *Guide*'s unwavering premise. It recognizes that we are individuals, with our own unique needs. Young people will feel valued, respected, and (dare I say this?) understood. They will stick with the *Guide*. It's like having someone around who offers great advice, and against whom a young person can test their own choices. Yet while it's pitched to young people, everyone

involved with them should read it. From any perspective, it's
engaging, useful, and deeply humane.

—Nathan Szajnberg, MD, clinical professor and research
fellow, San Francisco, New York, Jerusalem

Preface

This *Young Person's Guide* reflects my experience as a father and a psychiatrist. I am deeply, personally involved with young people—my three kids are adolescents, and I counsel public and private high school students in and around New York City. Sometimes I feel as though I live in young people's heads, trying to understand and help them cope with concerns that feel intense, immediate, and sometimes unique, but that are all part of a passage toward young adulthood. When I talk to young people, I tell them, "You're not alone. It's natural to think about what you think about. Just try to come out the other side in the best place you can." This book is a version of that advice. It's about how to make it through to realizing your best self. In practical terms, it's about developing habits to make all this easier over the next few years, habits that will sustain you even after you call yourself an adult.

In the introduction, I cite ten "tenets" (or principles) on which this book is based—for example, develop strong relationships, stay connected to a supportive community, take care of your body. I live by these tenets, and model them to my kids. These are not just ideas that it might be nice to follow. I strongly believe in them. I bring my kids up to believe in them. I monitor students whom I work with, and watch how they apply them and grow into more highly functioning individuals. I say "individuals" because the beauty of these tenets is that while they can be expressed in general terms, each person can apply them to fit their own situation. Taking care of your body is different for a member of the track team than it is for the captain of the chess team. Each, however, will choose foods and an exercise regimen that keep them fit and alert, and best suited to do what they love.

Of course, even while this *Guide* will be there for you, and offer real-world help to show you how to live these tenets, no one is suggesting that young people's lives are easy. During a single day, you may think about entering a sexual relationship (but what about STDs, and the emotional risks?); you may consider marijuana (but is it laced with PCP?); you may get distracted by influencers on social media (can you compete with their impossible body images?); you may wonder about your gender identity, the appropriateness of your friends, and whether you'll get into a good college. Your self-esteem is on the line, which entails your being accepted by the right peer group. You wrestle with doubts, which often you don't disclose. Finally, you wonder, "Should I talk to someone? Who?" These are real issues. This *Guide* acknowledges them. It will talk to you candidly about them. It will help you to begin to address them, based on where you are.

We all start from someplace. The point is to work toward the best place we can achieve. This takes work, which takes commitment. Don't rely on luck, or a last-minute fix. Take up these tenets and start living them—maybe not all at once, but at a pace you can sustain. Once you see results, and start believing in yourself, your pace will pick up. It will become self-reinforcing. I know because I see it happen. While we're all works in progress, it's the progress that makes us feel good. I wrote this *Guide* because feeling good about ourselves is entirely possible. That's the "wellness" in the *Guide*'s title. You can start now.

Introduction

This *Guide* grew out of the holistic health, wellness, and athletic program at a private school in New York, where the program seeks to help students to discover the best version of themselves. The *Guide* explores the program's ten tenets, which we will discuss in a moment. But first, what is "health" and "wellness"? The terms tend to blur around the edges, so we should recognize how each is important to developing young people's potential.

What is "health"? Wikipedia states that being "healthy" depends on our choices ("regular physical exercise and adequate sleep"), our luck (whether we have access to "necessary health-care services"), and our genetic makeup. Yet it also recognizes that beyond such factors, which largely confine "health" to the absence of disease, "health" has recently come to mean something more dynamic, less like a steady state than a type of resilience—a resource for coping with challenges when they throw us off base. In this view, "health" means that we adapt. We make the most of where we are now and may be in the future. The *Guide* follows this latter, more agile approach, and seeks to help students acquire the tools to stay strong (and effective!), even as circumstances change.

What is "wellness"? Wellness is a more complex, multidimensional concept than health. Rather than focusing on physicality, it integrates physical, intellectual, psychological, vocational, and social aspects of how we live. It sees these aspects as interdependent—you can't be a social success if your emotions shut down; you can't succeed in a vocation if your intellect is weak. Naturally, since each of us will place different emphases on these dimensions, "wellness" requires only that we find the right balance among them—what feels authentic to each of us in terms of our priorities and aspirations. Your wellness is not the same as mine. Still, none of this is easy. Wellness (however we experience it) requires that we develop good habits, enabling us to make the most of the dimensions of our lives that matter the most to us.

How do "health" and "wellness" intersect? By emphasizing good habits, wellness makes health easier to attain. But each concept has its own concerns and can help us discover the best version of ourselves depending on the context. The *Guide* recognizes the distinctiveness and complicated relationship of these two concepts.

What are the ten tenets of the health and wellness program? A "tenet" is a principle or belief, and thus a form of guidance. The program has adopted ten tenets, around which this *Guide* is structured:

1. You live in your body, so take care of it.
2. Good nutrition is essential for health.

3. Healthy habits strengthen you.
4. Self-reflection helps you find your way.
5. Core moral values improve your sense of self.
6. Healthy relationships are integral to your well-being.
7. Empathy is essential to caring about each other.
8. Building community helps you grow personally.
9. Nurturing a sound mind is important to physical health.
10. Making the most of good choices leads to a fulfilling life.

The *Guide* will help you think about how to apply these tenets to your own life. "What is good nutrition at my age?" "What relationships are healthy?" "How do I build community?" While the tenets may seem abstract (or at least unattainably lofty), you can make them part of your routine. Once you understand how they function in real-life, everyday terms, you can internalize them. Health and wellness should animate your life at school and beyond.

We expect that you will approach these tenets through practice and reflection, augmented by talking with people who are interested in your well-being. But as you consider them, think about (a) how they work together and (b) why they should become the basis for long-term health and wellness. Few of these tenets can be applied separately: self-reflection is necessary to maintaining good core values; empathy is necessary to cultivating relationships. The tenets' interdependence reflects the holistic approach of the program. Each chapter, explaining a particular tenet, will include questions for reflection and discussion—you won't start from ground zero. The point is to build awareness as you read.

Ultimately, the *Guide* will encourage you not to leave health and wellness to luck or chance, but to take responsibility for your psychological/physical well-being. What you do now affects you in the future. There is a seamlessness to life, so that we rarely perceive the unfolding consequences of what we do. Think of people who, later in life, sigh, "If only I had . . ." as they contemplate some mishap they might have avoided. But by developing an awareness of health and wellness, and by making it the basis of sound habits, you can better prepare for whatever comes next. You can integrate mental and physical well-being like the Romans did and maintain "a healthy mind in a healthy body." That advice has lasted for two thousand years, and it's still worth following.

Chapter 1

You live in your body, so take care of it

How do you take care of your body?

Before you can answer this question, you should think about the body's systems, which work together to help it to function. These systems operate autonomically, without our giving them much thought. Yet if we fail to care for them, we can do ourselves great damage.

Here is a summary of these systems:

Circulatory—The heart, blood, and blood vessels.

Respiratory—Primarily the lungs, which allow the body to take in oxygen and remove carbon dioxide.

Digestive—Organs such as the stomach and gall bladder, which convert food into energy and nutrients for the body.

Nervous—The brain, spinal cord, and nerves, through which the body receives sensory information and makes decisions.

Endocrine—A network of glands and organs that produce hormones which control many bodily functions, carrying information and instructions between cells.

Reproductive—Responsible for reproduction.

Musculoskeletal—Bones, muscles, joints, tendons, and ligaments, which allow us to move.

Excretory—Removes waste products.

Immune—Protects the body from infection, disease, and harmful substances.

Because these systems depend on each other, hormones from the endocrine system can affect the brain, altering your mood and sleep-wake cycle; the digestive system's ability (or inability) to metabolize milk will affect whether you get enough calcium to maintain strong bones.

Therefore, you should develop *habits* that help your body function properly, now and into the future. How you treat the body during young adulthood—while it is still developing—will have a profound effect on your physical and mental health as an adult.

Habits—If you don't have good habits (eating well, sleeping enough, getting exercise), you can form them. But first, what is a habit? It's a recurrent behavior that we don't consciously think about, which is acquired through frequent repetition. Habits are automatic, reflexive, spontaneous responses to given stimuli. Waiting for a red light is a habit (we see red, we stop). So is brushing our teeth after breakfast. Evolutionary theory suggests that habits developed to save us time and energy for more cognitively demanding activities.

How do habits develop? Basically, when some behavior results in a reward—for example, we cross the street safely—the brain builds a connection between that behavior and the resulting pleasure, so that the behavior becomes reflexive ("I always wear a helmet when I roller-blade"). The repeated link between the cue (going for a run), the action (filling the water bottle), and the reward (quenching a thirst) is how habits are created.

Thus, while we have all heard of "muscle memory" (Michael Jackson's dance routines, Kobe Bryant's moves), these memories are in the *brain* in the form of connections established (encoded, imprinted) over time.

Here are some good habits to get into (actually, they "get into" us by altering our brain pathways):

- Sleep enough (eight to ten hours a night), which helps support brain function, immune response, and recovery from fatigue.
- Exercise throughout the day to promote healthy circulation and maintain muscles.
- Eat well—reduce fats, avoid highly processed foods.
- Maintain a healthy weight.
- Pay attention to the *sources* of health information—check them out and avoid those that are dubious (like most "influencers," who are likely selling something).

Chapter III discusses habits in detail. But here, we emphasize the need to develop routines that support health and wellness.

Unfortunately, the downside of habit formation is that while we can develop good ones, we can just as easily fall into bad ones (smoking, alcohol addiction, nail biting, procrastination), since the behaviors that lead to such habits can also produce rewards (at least in the short term, and long enough for the behavior to become established). Once habits become encoded in our brain—beyond our ability to control them—they are *extremely* hard to break. It's important not to let bad habits develop. If you catch yourself biting your nails, or grabbing a cannabis gummy, just ask yourself, "Where is this leading?" "Do I have resources to stop on my own?" Get help if you need it (a team coach, the school nurse, your doctor).

Experts cite several strategies that can help break bad habits: avoid rationalizations ("Oh, everyone eats gummies"); monitor yourself ("How many gummies have I had this week?"); adopt safeguards (take a new route home to avoid your cannabis source); develop a group to hold you accountable; distract yourself (when you want a gummy, try yoga). Don't be embarrassed to share your concerns.

The bottom line about habit formation is that just as we create habits that help preserve our well-being, we can also damage our health irrevocably through inattention to what's best for us ("Hey, I've got plenty of time to quit smoking"). Your brain and body are still developing, so you should not do anything that can damage your bones, cause obesity, lower your cognitive ability, or predispose you to disease later in life. The time for healthy habits is *now*—not later, when it could be difficult or impossible to reverse the damage.

Choices—Research shows that habit governs about 40 percent of our everyday behavior. That's huge. Still, human beings are not automatons. We make choices that *lead* to habits and that affect our well-being. But how do we make the right choices? We exercise our best, most informed judgment. We consider our options, and never act impetuously (bad choices can be hard to correct). We weigh the risks and calculate the relationship between the cost of some choice and its benefits. We consider the impact on those around us.

Young people tend to act before they've thought through the available options. For example, a sixteen-year-old may choose to spend the summer at baseball camp, not stopping to think that a creative writing course might also be fun, or going on a trek in Yosemite, or even helping people learn English. It's important just to slow down. In *Thinking, Fast and Slow*, Nobel Prize-winner Daniel Kahneman makes a distinction between types of actions that are amenable to fast thinking—say, choosing your socks in the morning—and those that require slower, deliberative mental processes. The latter might include compiling a guide to computer accessories, or—in your case—choosing the best option for how to spend the summer; what courses to choose in the fall; whether to break up with someone after a fight. Most important choices require the input of time, and a consideration of a lot of "what-ifs." After enough what-ifs, you can finally decide "then that." Think of thinking slowly as a series of what-ifs: "What are the consequences of choosing basketball camp over a trek in the Andes?" "Do I want to spend the summer with a bunch of basketball nerds, or do I want to experience a culture that is new and strange?" "If I am really interested in exercising to the max, will I possibly injure myself?" What-ifs are a kind of trial run in your mind, where you examine the consequences from a variety of perspectives before making up your mind. It's really a type of critical thinking based on assessing all the data you can aggregate. You could, in fact, make it a habit.

If nothing else, remember that choices made in the moment (like taking drugs or having sex) can have a lasting impact. One overdose, and we might never recover. Also, remember that the *process* of evaluating risk changes over time. Adults have more experience to back them up. They may have access to sources of information that you don't—for example, friends who are an expert in some area that could inform their decision-making. The point is just to be careful—there's a lot of room to mess up and, of course, you don't want to.

Common sense—We should learn to listen to our body: eat when we're hungry, rest when we're tired, stop pushing when we feel pain (exercising "through" pain can be disastrous, and is only for pro athletes under medical supervision). We should put down our phones and socialize, get exercise, experience the world. But we should also resist pressure to experiment with drugs and alcohol, since these can have lasting detrimental effects. We should think before engaging in sex (we can get hurt, and we can hurt others), and we should always practice safe sex to avoid getting an STD (talk to an RN or a doctor). In America, male teenagers start having sex, on average, at around 16.8 years of age. For females, it's around 17.2 years. Research shows that, nonetheless, most young people feel that they started too early.

We will talk later about choosing friends and romantic partners. But here, we stress the importance of thinking through the consequences of the choices you can make that potentially affect your body. "Do I want to go out for football, where I might get a concussion, or should I try for a spot on the swim team?" "Do I want that extra piece of chocolate cake, or should I choose a peach?" "Should I take my bike on a rain-slicked road, or wait for the bus?" Choices are endless, but in most cases, thinking them through just requires the application of your common sense unclouded by peer pressure, whims, or desires of the moment. You can seek advice if you're unsure. It's still easier than making the wrong, possibly damaging choice.

Assessing the risks, cost/benefit analyses—There are quantifiable scenarios where the risk is low but the impact is high. In these cases, there may be only a 10 percent chance of an accident . . . but if it happens, you could break your neck. So, assess your risk realistically. Don't let your immediate impulses cloud your judgment ("Oh, I'm careful on my bike, so who cares about the rain?"). The best choices are usually informed by experience, and we may think we have more than we do. Choice is a balancing act, so give yourself enough time to learn about what goes into any choice before you make it. Assess all the risks, and *then* choose.

Likewise, there's another common scenario called cost/benefit analysis. Here, you don't weigh the quantum of risk against various potential outcomes. Instead, you take the known costs and weigh them against the likely benefits—if the costs outweigh the benefits, then you should likely discard the project. If going to basketball camp will produce only a marginal benefit in your performance ("I just don't have the height"), why incur the cost of missing a summer of seeing friends, taking fun day trips, and maybe taking that writing course at a local college?

Consider the effect on other people—This *Guide* makes the point, again and again, that whatever we do affects other people, just as what they do affects us. It's part of living in a habitable community that everyone treats everyone carefully, and with respect. When we make choices, they should reflect our understanding of how they'll ripple through other people's lives. Do they limit resources that other people should be able to access? Do they contribute to disorder or uncertainty, and make life less bearable for those around us? Just because we *can* choose one option over another, doesn't mean that we *should*. We need to act fairly and conscientiously because, in the final analysis, how we affect others will come back around to us. We should leave space for people so that they feel comfortable taking our needs into consideration. We don't want to crowd them and limit their impulse toward generosity.

We should not to be so concerned with our immediate self-interest that we miss the big picture—which includes everyone else, now and into the future. Our choices should be informed by a sense of communality, since we are part of the community.

Use AI, but do not rely on it—While AI is everywhere, and using it is inevitable, we shouldn't let it do our thinking for us. It's fine to ask AI a question and get an initial leg up on a problem. But relying on it stifles creativity. It turns thought processes into an extension of an algorithm. It displaces personality (who wants to be homogenized into what everyone else has ever said?). It promotes intellectual laziness that can hamper us as life gets more complex. Instead, we should practice dealing with complexity. If we're rushed, we should slow down enough to think for ourselves.

Don't waste time on social media—While it's fun to follow your friends on Instagram, and pick up on the latest TikTok threads, you can easily find yourself absorbed for hours on social media. It can become a distraction and even an obsession. You can also subject yourself to misinformation from so-called influencers, who are intent on making money off everyone else's credulity. You can develop distorted ideas about "perfect" body types that can have real physical implications. Limit the time that you spend on these platforms. Also, be careful about what you post—it can come back around at you and be hugely embarrassing. You may think that if you're not totally involved, you're missing out, but you are just protecting your personal head-space. The bottom line is that what you do on social media is not trivial. Like all the other choices you make, deciding how often to sign on, what to believe, and what to say are matters of consequence. They can affect how you see the world, how you see yourself, and how the world sees you.

Mind/body/disposition—The mind and body are parts of a single entity. *The one affects the other*: if you are anxious, your eating habits can suffer; if you're tired, your thought processes become foggy. Thus, in caring for the body, it is crucial to care for yourself psychologically. Just as you wouldn't let a wound fester, don't ignore anxiety, depression, and related conditions.

Depression in young people is a serious medical condition that can make it hard to function normally. It's more than just feeling sad for a few days, or being moody. Rather, it's intense sadness, hopelessness, anger, or frustration that lasts much longer. You turn inward, and may avoid people, which just makes the condition worse. It's hard to enjoy life or even get through the day. The future seems like more of the same.

The National Institute of Mental Health (NIMH) offers guidance to teens who may suffer from depression. It suggests you ask yourself these questions to see if you should be concerned.

- Do I often feel sad, anxious, worthless, or even "empty"?
- Have I lost interest in activities that I used to enjoy?
- Do I get easily frustrated, irritable, or angry?
- Do I find myself withdrawing from friends and family?
- Are my grades dropping?
- Have my eating or sleeping habits changed?
- Have I experienced any fatigue or memory loss?
- Have I thought about suicide or harming myself?

NIMH notes that depression looks different for everyone. You might have many of the symptoms listed above, or just a few. But the point is that you don't have to face these symptoms alone. Help is available. In the most extreme cases, you can call or text the Suicide and Crisis Lifeline at 988 or chat at 988lifeline.org. Here are some other steps that NIMH recommends.

- Talk to a trusted adult about how you've been feeling.
- Ask your doctor about options for professional help.

- Try to spend time with family or friends, even if you don't feel like it.
- Stay active and exercise, even if it's just going for a walk (physical activity releases chemicals in your brain that can help you feel better).
- Try to keep a regular sleep schedule.
- Eat healthy foods.

Through a combination of self-awareness, common sense, and reaching out to others (including professionals), you can get better.

Stress management—There is so much to do. So much to think about. There never seems like enough time to do it all, let alone do it well. But if you're always stressed out, chances are you won't do anything well. There may be physical consequences, since we know that stress can cause insomnia, headaches, decreased immunity, skin rashes, reduced sex drive, reduced appetite, and an array of other problems. So, if you feel stressed, then slow down. Try to determine what can be put off until a later time. *Establish priorities.* Let off steam by tossing a ball around, or running. You might also listen to music, or do a crossword puzzle. You can do yoga. Never retreat into smoking or drugs, which will only damage your body.

But apart from alleviating stress, try to prevent it in the first place. For example, if you have a paper due in two weeks, don't start it the night before. Start it a week before. When you come back to it, you'll have time to think and be creative. You'll spot errors. You won't crash to get something in on time, and you won't worry—before and after you submit it—about whether it's your best work. The fact is that a lot of stress can

11

be avoided just by managing time and the demands on us. If you feel stressed, it's okay to explain that you do, and to decline requests that will take even more of your time.

Naturally, the sources of stress vary. Stress can result from conflict with your parents (or conflict between your parents that affects you); from a relationship; from expectations that didn't work out ("I was sure I'd get into an Ivy—now I've disappointed everyone"). These types of stresses can lead to grief and even depression, since we may feel helpless to deal with them. In these instances, as in any situation that seems too big to handle, try to find help. It's important not to let stress persist, whatever the cause.

Drugs, smoking, and alcohol—Drugs can damage your brain's development. Smoking can harm your lungs, your heart, and your immune system—as well as creating an ugly habit that's extremely hard to break. Alcohol (except perhaps an occasional beer or glass of wine) can lead to long-term habits that can cause liver disease. In the short term, it can muddle your thinking. So don't try any of these. If you are tempted to experiment, then remind yourself that there are dozens of other ways to have fun or blow off steam. Besides, it's illegal in all fifty states to use tobacco, alcohol, and cannabis/marijuana if you're a minor.

When you feel tempted, you may think, "Oh, it's just marijuana—I'd never go near the hard stuff." But in some instances, marijuana can be a "gateway" drug that leads to harder drugs. You may also think that marijuana and some other drugs are prescribed to address certain medical conditions. But that's just the point—they're *prescribed* by professionals in highly controlled situations. That's not your situation.

But suppose you're at a party, and everyone's passing a joint around. Or suppose they're all drinking. The social pressure is intense. You don't want to seem like a square, but you also don't want to do anything that could harm you. What do you do? How do you gracefully decline a joint or a drink? You might say something like, "I don't like getting high, because I have more fun when I'm not." Or maybe, if it's true, "I'm biking home later, so I've got to remain alert." The point is not to show disapproval, but just to demonstrate that your personal circumstances don't lend themselves to indulgence right now. No fuss. Just politely decline.

Takeaways—The body is a complex mechanism that needs close attention. In the case of young people, proper care now—when the body is still developing—will mean fewer physical (and related mental) problems later. It's crucial to develop good habits and avoid bad ones. Of course, none of this is easy (just think of the peer pressure pushing you in directions that you may not want to go). It takes a conscious effort, supported by reliable information and by people that you trust. If you embark on caring for your body now, you'll be happier as you grow into it.

Follow-up questions to ask yourself and to discuss:

- Do I have habits that may be harmful, and do I know how I can work on breaking them?
- Am I willing to talk about my concerns with people that I trust, or do I keep my concerns bottled up?

- Do I make informed choices, and measure the likely risks before choosing?
- Do I feel anxious or depressed, and am I seeking help?
- Do I manage stress effectively by taking breaks, and do I arrange my life so that I can avoid stress whenever possible?
- Do I dislike my body image in ways that cause me to restrict my food consumption to unnaturally low levels? If so, am I seeking help with this condition?
- Have I been able to resist drugs, smoking, and alcohol? Do I know how to find support so that I can resist them?

Further reading

Davis, Martha. *The Relaxation and Stress Reduction Workbook.* New Harbinger Publications, 2019.

Friedberg, Ahron, MD, with Sandra Sherman. *Life Studies in Psychoanalysis: Faces of Love.* Routledge, 2023.

Haidt, Jonathan. *The Anxious Generation: How the Great Rewiring of Childhood is Causing an Epidemic of Mental Illness.* Penguin, 2024.

Kahneman, Daniel. *Thinking, Fast and Slow.* Farrar, Straus and Giroux, 2013.

Stock, Braxton. *Understanding Gender Identity.* Dedicated Publishing, 2023.

White, Melody. *Yoga Guide for Beginners: 101 Poses and Sequences for Strength, Flexibility, and Mindfulness.* CreateSpace, 2018.

Chapter II

Good nutrition is essential for health

Everyone knows that good food is important. But what is "good" food, and how much of it should we eat? Here's where good nutrition comes in, which is defined as eating the right foods, in the right balance, in the right quantities to ensure your health and growth. It involves *conscious* eating, where you decide what's good based on criteria that transcend how something tastes. "That chocolate cake is *good*" doesn't fit the criteria. Good nutrition is the opposite of eating on impulse; or just to satisfy your hunger; or to alleviate stress; or to get a sugar rush. It's intellectually motivated, supported by sufficient willpower.

Your decisions won't necessarily be like someone else's, since your body type and degree of activity may differ from theirs. An athlete, for example, requires more calories from different sources (mainly carbs) than a chess player. Their basal metabolic rate (the number of calories needed to maintain homeostasis, or the equilibrium among various physiological processes) will also likely be different, since muscle mass requires more energy to maintain than does other tissue. Good nutrition involves a matrix of individualized decisions that lead you to make optimal choices.

Ultimately, if good food choices transition into good habits—in other words, into your lifestyle—then "conscious" eating becomes natural. You won't have to think about it much.

Of course, some foods are generally regarded as "good." They're high in protein, for example, and are good sources of vitamins and minerals. But you still need to decide how much of any food to eat, as well as how much food overall so that you don't risk obesity (currently a national epidemic). You should choose foods that support your gut's microbiome. You can even choose foods to support the growth of hair and nails, reduce inflammation, and counteract skin dehydration.

When you make good nutrition a habit, you eat what's healthy for *you*. You learn what works, though of course, you can always adjust ("I'm running the 15K this weekend, so I'll load up on carbs a few days in advance"). The point is to get to know your body and the nutritional regimen that will keep you healthy, strong, and growing.

One way to begin a personal food regimen is to focus on portion control and lifestyle changes. Perhaps you won't eat out as much. That way, you can limit your portions and see what goes into your food (how much salt? how much butter?). Maybe you learn to cook your favorite dishes in right-sized portions. You're not exactly on a diet or counting calories, but you're taking sensible steps reflecting your own nutritional requirements.

You should also consider your diet's secondary effects— apart from maintaining your weight, muscle mass, and a healthy biome, it plays a role in your ability to focus. With the right nutrition, you won't seek out so-called energy boosters, which can have harmful side effects. You won't need eight cups of coffee a day, or binge on energy bars that are close to candy.

You're eating for now and for the future. If, for example, you don't get enough calcium, your bones will not be as strong in your thirties, forties, and beyond. They could fracture. If you eat too many sugary foods, you could predispose yourself to diabetes. Consider good nutrition as a type of insurance— not just for optimal development during your adolescence, but for your durability as an adult.

Here is some information to get you started.

The food groups—The US Department of Agriculture (USDA) has elaborate guidelines on how to structure your food intake, the *Dietary Guidelines for Americans*, which is cited below under Further Reading. Still, it's useful in broad outline, and suggests that we consume food from each of five food groups:

- Fruits
- Vegetables (dark green, red, and orange; beans/peas/ lentils; starchy; and all the others)
- Grains

- Protein foods (fish, meat, poultry, eggs, nuts, seeds, and soy)
- Dairy (milk, yogurt, cheese)

These categories are somewhat arbitrary, since there is protein in dairy, grains, vegetables, and even some fruits (like guava, avocado, apricots, and raisins). However, while animal protein is "complete" on a molecular level, the protein in nuts, grains, or vegetables is not. If you avoid food groups that include animal protein, you'll need to investigate the right combinations of foods that will supply the protein you need. Mixing beans and grains, for example, is a common strategy, but you'll need to do some research when designing your own diet.

Choosing foods. There are some common ground rules for getting the most from our diet. Here are some basic considerations:

Nutrient-dense foods—The USDA encourages us to choose foods in their most nutrient-dense forms, and to keep added sugars and saturated fats below 10 percent of our total calorie intake. You can think of a nutrient-dense food by comparing nonfat plain yogurt to chocolate ice cream (both contain milk protein, but while a cup of yogurt contains 13 grams/80 calories, the ice cream contains 5 grams/286 calories).

Think for a moment. While Cocoa Puffs and Frosted Flakes are made from grain (one of the five food groups), they are so loaded with sugar (over 25 percent by weight in Cocoa Puffs) that they cannot count as nutrient-dense. A bowl of oatmeal or unsweetened wheat germ is vastly better. Not coincidentally, sugary cereals are highly processed, which means that they have been significantly altered from their natural state by an array of additives that may include fats, starches, sugars, salt, hydrogenated oils, and chemicals that are hard to pronounce. The less processing, the more likely a food is to be nutrient-dense rather than just a source of empty calories. Also, the less likely it is to become addictive—research demonstrates that big food companies deliberately design foods so that we crave more and more (remember the famous Lay's potato chip ad, "Betcha can't eat just one"?).

When you choose foods, pay attention to a basic calculation: what's *really* in that food relative to what I need? Then go with foods where the calculation is in your favor. You can still eat foods where it's not so favorable, but—as with everything you eat—exercise moderation.

Portion control—Suppose you're a chocoholic. You can eat an entire eight-ounce bag of Hershey's Kisses (152 calories/ oz) starting from the time you wake up ("Hey, what's a few with my oatmeal?") to the time you need a snack before bed ("There's just a few left, so I might as well finish them"). But there are better ways of getting 1,200 calories. Just before your next craving, set aside three or four kisses and put the bag away. Effectively, you're limiting the quantity that you'll consume, which is the essence of portion control. Former president Barack Obama famously took seven almonds with him when he returned to his study after dinner to prepare for the next day.

If, instead of chocolate, you love steak, try sharing your next ribeye with someone. You still get to enjoy it but, again, you're limiting the portion to what's more reasonable in terms of fat and calories. Maybe even make Chinese beef with broccoli, where the steak goes even further, and the new taste sensation would be interesting.

You don't have to give up what you like in order to eat a "healthy" diet, though you should make adjustments that keep you from overeating. They're part of conscious eating.

Calories—An active teenage boy needs about 2,600–3,200 calories a day, while an active teenage girl needs about 2,200–2,400 calories. These amounts will vary with your energy expenditure, height, and weight, as well as your metabolic rate (how fast you burn calories). *What's important is that your calories be derived from nutrient-dense foods and that you eat a balance of foods from an array of food groups—fruits, vegetables, grains, protein, and dairy. You can adjust to your specific needs based on your body type and activity level.*

You're not on a "diet" unless a doctor puts you on one! The USDA's general patterns for daily food consumption (designed to help us meet our nutritional needs) can help you eat *a balanced diet, right-sized for you.* After a while, you will naturally choose the right foods in sensible quantities. The point is to integrate eating into a healthy lifestyle that includes exercise and ways of relieving stress.

Here are some basics:

Protein. Your body needs proteins (amino acid building blocks) for several reasons:

- Proteins help to build and repair tissue.
- Red blood cells contain a protein (hemoglobin) that carries oxygen throughout the body.

- Enzymes are proteins that aid in digestion and other critical processes in the body.
- Valuable hormones like insulin are proteins.

The amount of protein teenagers need depends on their age, sex, body weight, stage of development, and activity level. In general, boys between the ages of fourteen and eighteen need 52 grams per day. Girls need 46. But these amounts can vary, so talk to someone knowledgeable about the amount that's right for you.

You would get more than enough protein if you had an egg and a bowl of oatmeal for breakfast, a burger with skim milk for lunch, and lentil soup, a black bean salad, and whole wheat bread for dinner. Once you know how much protein is in a serving of food, and how much protein you need, you can design your meals accordingly.

But no matter how *much* protein you need, it's important to determine *how best to get it*. This is because not all protein is the same. The body makes some non-essential amino acids, but essential amino acids must come from food, and those foods differ in what proteins they supply. Animal products and soy contain all the essential amino acids (so they're called "complete" proteins). Most plant foods, like beans, nuts, and grains, are incomplete. Vegans and vegetarians combine incomplete proteins to create a meal with all the essential amino acids. They would pick from one group (beans and nuts) and combine it with another (grains).

The point is to make sure that whatever your diet, you get enough protein to sustain your body's development and its ability to function. The emphasis here is on *your* body, since bodies differ across an array of parameters.

It's also important to evaluate the protein sources you choose in terms of their nutrient density. A Big Mac contains 26 grams of protein, which sounds like a lot. But once you consider the high fat content, you might choose a different option. Likewise, protein bars often have 10 or 12 grams of protein from soy, but if they are covered in chocolate, they will likely have a high number of calories from sugar.

Sodium/salt. While salt is necessary for life, too much sodium can lead to high blood pressure, heart disease, and stroke. You should avoid too much sodium—no more than 2,300 mg per day (about a teaspoon of salt). The problem for American food consumers is that salt is added to almost everything—you may not taste it, but it's there. For example, a slice of white bread has about 175 mg of salt. If you have a couple of pieces for breakfast, and then a sandwich for lunch, you're already up to 700 mg before you eat anything else for breakfast (like cornflakes, with 200 mg/cup) or put anything on your sandwich (like Swiss cheese, with 50+ mg/oz). A typical slice of pizza has over 600 mg. Chinese dumplings dipped in soy sauce (almost 900 mg/tablespoon) could send you close to the limit.

As we discuss below, it's important to read the labels on foods—when there is a label. For example, chain restaurants in many states and localities must provide information on sodium content where foods contain levels considered to be high. In New York City, you can look for a warning icon next to offending items. But the best way to avoid too much sodium is just to avoid highly processed foods. Even if a label says "reduced sodium," there can still be too much for a healthy diet.

When you cook at home, skip some of the added salt and experiment with spices. After a while, you'll get used to food that's less salty (and you may get to love the interesting results you get by experimenting with spices and spice blends—just make sure that the "blends" do not contain salt, as do most commercial mixtures sold as chili powder). You could even try making your own salsa, emphasizing the peppers and onions and reducing the salt.

Remember, just be sensible. Learn what to avoid (most of the time), and find stuff that you like and that's good for you. Then make eating the good stuff a habit.

Fats—saturated, unsaturated, trans (or hydrogenated) fats, and cholesterol. The chemistry of fats is complicated. First, it's important to limit consumption of saturated fat (the kind in butter, lard, marbled red meat, bacon, chicken with the skin on, and full-fat dairy products). Cheeses like cheddar, cream cheese, and brie also contain these fats in high concentrations. It's okay for most people to have such fats now and then, but eating too much can lead to high blood pressure, stroke, and heart conditions. You're eating now with an eye on the future.

Trans fats are extremely unhealthy. They are a type of processed food that is created when liquid oils (such as corn oil) are turned into solid fats, like shortening or margarine, by altering their chemistry through hydrogenation. The good news, however, is that the Food and Drug Administration (FDA) banned most uses of these fats, though small amounts still exist in some foods.

Cholesterol is a lipid, like fat, but it occurs only in animals. Yet unlike other fats, it cannot be metabolized for energy, though it is useful in building cells and making hormones. If we consume too much cholesterol, it can cause plaque buildup in our arteries, leading to heart disease and stroke. This is why we're told to limit the eggs we consume, since they are high in cholesterol.

In general, it's better to consume monounsaturated fat from olives, avocados, and nuts. Some fish (like salmon, tuna, mackerel, herring, and sardines) are high in omega-3 fatty acids that *support* heart health. Again, it's important to read food labels, which are required to list the amounts of saturated and unsaturated fats, as well as cholesterol.

In practical terms, try cooking with olive oil instead of butter. Eat fish high in omega-3. When you buy dairy products, go for the low-fat or nonfat options. Choose skinless chicken breasts and ground beef that is at least 90 percent lean. Ground turkey is often 95 percent or more lean.

Just remember that highly saturated fats and cholesterol can build up in the body and harden your arteries. That means that they will be less able to carry blood (and oxygen) to your organs. This can result in shortness of breath, heart attacks, and stroke. You're building your body now for the future. If you take reasonable steps now to limit fat—and you continue taking them—you'll be better off as you get older.

Fiber. Fiber is an indigestible substance found in (unprocessed) foods that can reduce the risk of colon cancer and hemorrhoids, lower the risk of heart disease, prevent spikes in blood sugar, and help prevent constipation. Whole grains (as opposed to refined flour with the germ extracted and polishings removed) are a good source of fiber—so try eating whole wheat toast for breakfast. Avocados, almonds, brussels sprouts, broccoli, oatmeal, beans, apples, and blueberries are all high in fiber. So is unpolished (brown) rice.

Refined sugar. Sugar occurs naturally. It's in fruit (fructose), grain (barley contains maltose), and even milk (lactose). But nutritional problems arise when naturally occurring sugars are refined, removing their trace nutrients and otherwise chemically changing them. For example, high fructose corn syrup (HFCS), a type of refined sugar frequently added to soft drinks, canned foods, baked goods, and dairy products, has been linked to obesity, diabetes, inflammation, tooth decay, and liver disease.

You can't just assume that "sugar is sugar," and that one type of sugar (say, in a peach) is the same as the next (say, in Oreos). Unless you read a food's label, you may not even realize that HFCS is present. You may not stop to think that other refined sugars are present, for example, in juices with nice pictures of fruit on the bottle. Unless the product says "100 percent juice" (or 100 percent whatever), you should find out the actual percentage of added sugar. Jams and jellies are usually 50 percent (or more) refined sugar.

The USDA's *Guidelines* recommend limiting added sugar to no more than 10 percent of our total calorie intake. But that seems overly generous to the sugar refiners. For example, if you consume 2,000 calories a day, then that works out to 200 calories from sugar, equal to about 12 teaspoons. Presumably, you could get along with less.

Weirdly, there was a period in the seventeenth and eighteenth centuries when sugar was regarded as medicine. People ate as much as they could, until it was discovered that too much sugar caused tooth decay. Now the problem is obesity, which adversely affects longevity and one's quality of life. According to the Food Research & Action Center, 39.6 percent of US adults are obese. This is in addition to the 31.6 percent who are overweight, and 7.7 percent who are severely obese. The bottom line is that refined sugar, like all highly processed foods, just isn't good for you.

Vitamins and minerals. Teenagers need the same vitamins and minerals as adults, but some are especially important:

- *Iron*—Helps develop strong bones and maintain energy, and is especially important for girls, who lose iron through menstruation. Iron is found in animal sources like meat, eggs, and fish, and in plant sources like whole grains, dark leafy greens, beans, and dried fruits. Failure to get enough iron can result in anemia.

- *Zinc*—Supports growth, sexual maturation, and a strong immune system. Also important for treating acne. Low levels can reduce cognitive function. Good sources include meat and poultry.

- *Calcium*—Necessary for strong bones. A high-sodium diet causes the body to lose calcium, as does excessive dieting. Milk products are the best source.

- *Vitamin D*—Helps the body absorb calcium, which is important for strong bones and a healthy immune system. The best source is regular exposure to sunlight, although oily fish such as sardines, mackerel, and salmon are also good. Most milk is "fortified" with Vitamin D.

- *Vitamin A*—Supports healthy skin and vision, and is essential for growth and tissue repair. Carrots and pumpkin are great sources.
- *Vitamin B6*—Low levels can contribute to acne, mood swings, and sugar cravings. Good sources include meat, poultry, and fish.
- *Vitamin B12*—Helps form red blood cells, which carry oxygen throughout the body. May also help maintain energy levels. Good sources include meat, fish, poultry, and dairy.
- *Vitamin C*—Helps support the immune system, absorb iron, and build collagen (which provides structure and support to many tissues and organs). Keeps teeth, bones, and gums healthy. Citrus fruits are an excellent source.

Check with a nurse, doctor, nutritionist, or dietitian to see if your diet provides enough of these and other essential vitamins and minerals. This is especially necessary if you are a vegetarian/vegan and need to rely on non-animal sources of iron. If your diet is insufficient, you should consider taking a supplement. But if everyone agrees that you are eating well, you do not need to dose yourself to achieve elevated levels of any vitamin or mineral. Some people take a daily multivitamin-mineral supplement just for "insurance."

Caffeine. Caffeine is popular because it keeps us awake. It's a type of energy-booster. But according to the American Academy of Pediatrics, adolescents aged twelve to eighteen should limit their caffeine intake to less than 100 mg per day (or just about the amount in one eight-ounce cup of coffee). This is because teenagers' bodies are more sensitive to caffeine than adults', and larger amounts can have such negative effects as nervousness, irritability, nausea, sleep impairment, anxiety, and even high blood pressure. So, monitor your coffee intake.

Some drinks other than coffee have significant amounts of caffeine. A twelve-ounce can of Diet Coke has 46 mg—drink two of those, and you're near the recommended limit. A twelve-ounce can of Red Bull has 84 mg. But that's still modest compared to other energy drinks: Celsius Heat, Bang, and Rockstar Xdurance all have more than four times than that per can.

So, how do you get an energy boost without consuming caffeine? Drinking water in the morning can help by increasing the oxygen in your bloodstream. Eating a balanced diet can help. You can also eat foods with a low glycemic (sugar) index, such as most fruits and vegetables, beans, lentils, dried seeds, and minimally processed grains. These provide a steady release of energy as compared to foods that are high in sugar—the latter provide a "sugar rush," followed by an energy letdown. Apart from food, exercise and sufficient sleep are also energy boosters.

If discipline isn't your style, it's okay to occasionally indulge. There's that old saying about "everything in moderation," which also applies to your food choices. Just remember that there's also that other old saying, "you are what you eat," which means that too much junk food is a bad idea. It's up to you. Your brain and body are still developing, so keep that in mind.

The microbiome—Research demonstrates that highly processed foods can cause a temporary spike in blood sugar. When this occurs, you feel a rush of energy, only to quickly experience a letdown. This amounts to a mood swing, where the bottom can feel almost like depression. It's better to eat foods that release their sugars at a steady rate and don't cause disorienting spikes. Sugary drinks can have effects on energy levels that are like those of highly processed foods.

Processed foods, which lack basic nutrients and can be full of artificial chemicals, may also interfere with the gut-brain connection. The gut is home to millions of bacteria (the "microbiome") that influence the production of chemical substances that carry messages from the gut to the brain. These substances include dopamine and serotonin. Dopamine helps nerve cells communicate with each other and plays a role in many bodily functions. It is sometimes called the "feel-good" hormone because it can create feelings of pleasure, satisfaction, and motivation. It also affects the sleep/wake cycle, which in turn affects one's mood. Serotonin carries messages between nerve cells throughout the body. It is a natural mood booster, and is involved in regulating emotions like anger fear, and stress. Low serotonin levels have been linked to depression.

On the other hand, nutritionally dense foods promote the growth of bacteria that positively affect the production of dopamine and serotonin, among other important chemicals.

When viewed from the perspective of the gut-brain connection, good nutrition takes on a whole new objective: ensuring that you don't interfere with the production of chemicals that help you maintain a good mood.

Even apart from conditions like anxiety and depression, the microbiome plays a major role in digestion and the extraction of nutrients from foods. It affects brain development and nerve signaling. Imbalances in the microbiome have been linked to inflammatory diseases, cancer, and diabetes. These are all major concerns. To maintain a healthy microbiome, eat plenty of plant fiber, as well as good fats like omega-3 and unsaturated fats like those in avocados.

The bottom line on eating is that when you choose foods, go for the least processed—usually, these have the fewest chemicals and the least added salt. They contain little or no added sugars. The fiber has not been polished off or refined away. The amount of saturated fat is low or nonexistent.

Read the label—How do you know what's really in foods? Read the labels, like this one for wattleseeds from the Australian acacia tree:

From the label, we can determine that this is a nutrient-dense food. A serving satisfies a whopping 40 percent of the protein requirement of someone on a 2,000-calorie diet. It contributes a high percentage of the person's daily requirement for magnesium, calcium, and iron. The amount of dietary fiber is *huge*, and the fat content is low. On the other hand, don't rely on wattle seeds as a source of Vitamin D—there is none.

Almost all packaged foods must have food labels. But if a food is unpackaged and without a label, it's still possible to determine its nutrient density. Just look up the food online and examine the sugar, fat, and nutrient content. For example,

Nutrition Facts

Serving size	100 grams

Amount Per Serving

Calories 280

	% Daily Value*
Total Fat 6g	**8%**
Saturated Fat 0.8g	**4%**
Trans Fat 0g	
Polyunsaturated Fat 3.27g	
Monounsaturated Fat 1.5g	
Cholesterol 0mg	**0%**
Sodium 100mg	**4%**
Total Carbohydrate 10g	**4%**
Dietary Fiber 54g	**193%**
Total Sugars 0g	
Includes 0g Added Sugars	**0%**
Protein 20g	**40%**
Vitamin D 0mcg	0%
Calcium 419mg	30%
Iron 6mg	35%
Potassium 961mg	20%
Magnesium 243mg	60%

*The % Daily Value (DV) tells you how much a nutrient in a serving of food contributes to a daily diet. 2,000 calories a day is used for general nutrition advice.

if you look up "nutrients in broccoli," you'll get a full list—including trace nutrients that you hadn't even thought of.

Superfoods—You've probably heard of "superfoods," which are said to boost an already healthy diet. While such claims should be taken with a (figurative) grain of salt, there is still some truth to the idea that certain foods are so nutritious that we should include them in our diet on a regular basis. In October 2022, Harvard Medical School issued a bulletin (cited in the Further Reading section at the end of this chapter) listing ten of these foods.

- *Berries*—high in fiber and disease-fighting substances
- *Fish*—a good source of protein and omega-3 fatty acids
- *Leafy greens*—good source of vitamins A and C, calcium, and phytochemicals (health-boosting chemicals produced by plants)
- *Nuts*—good source of plant protein and monounsaturated fats (a possible factor in reducing the risk of heart disease)
- *Olive oil*—good source of vitamin E and monounsaturated fats
- *Whole grains*—good source of fiber B vitamins and phytonutrients
- *Yogurt*—good source of calcium and protein, as well as probiotic bacteria (which help defend the body from harmful bacteria)
- *Cruciferous vegetables*—broccoli, brussels sprouts, cauliflower, cabbage, kale, among others, and an

excellent source of fiber, vitamins, and important phytochemicals
- *Legumes*—excellent source of plant-based proteins
- *Tomatoes*—high in vitamin C and a chemical shown to reduce the risk of prostate cancer

Food is not medicine. It cannot cure or prevent disease. But some foods are better for us than others. The ten foods listed here, while not necessarily "better" than everything in most people's diets, are certainly very good and better than *some* things in our diets. Even if you choose a few ("I don't like broccoli, but I love blueberries"), you've upped your game.

It's also true that Harvard's list hardly precludes other superfoods from other lists. Avocados, green tea, sweet potatoes, dark chocolate, and even spices like turmeric and herbs like ginger all have their advocates. This lengthening list just demonstrates that so many foods are good for us, provided we avoid the obvious culprits like their highly processed relatives.

Diets and supplements—We've all heard of various diets that are supposed to keep us fit and healthy: Mediterranean, paleo, ketogenic, vegetarian, vegan, intermittent fasting, and Atkins (to name a few). They all have their strong points. They all require work. But mostly, unless you cannot tolerate certain foods and must be on a strict diet (for example, if you're lactose-intolerant), it's unnecessary to follow a formulaic eating pattern. Just eat nutrient-dense foods, and limit foods that may be harmful down the road. Limit your intake of salt, refined sugar, saturated fat, and cholesterol. After a while, you can develop your own diet ("I feel better if I eat lots of fiber for breakfast—it sets me up for the day"). You know your own body best.

Of course, you shouldn't skip meals. Or binge. Just eat a variety of foods in sensible quantities. Fruits and vegetables in a variety of colors (red, orange, yellow, green, blue) will ensure you get enough antioxidants (substances that reduce inflammation and cell damage and support disease prevention).

If you eat sensibly, you won't need all the supplements found online and in health food stores—like powdered soy protein, whey protein, powdered fruit and vegetable pills, and fish oil capsules. You won't need to dose yourself with vitamins and minerals—you'll get enough naturally. If you uncomplicate eating and stick to the basics, you'll be fine. But if you have questions, talk to someone reliable—a nurse, a coach, or a nutritionist.

Body image and eating disorders—Because body image is so important to our self-esteem, and to our estimation of how other people perceive us, we may try to restrict our food consumption to unnaturally low levels. We equate "thinner" with "better." The worst part is when this effort becomes a habit that we can no longer control. Bulimia and anorexia are the result. If they become chronic, they may require intense medical intervention *to save our lives*. At the very least, they can upset our endocrine system and reduce our bone density (leading to osteoporosis as we age). If you notice that you're not eating the way you have in the recent past, don't hide it. Talk to a nurse or to your parents. Get help early. The sooner these conditions are addressed, the less risk they pose. The National Eating Disorders Association (https://www.nationaleatingdisorders.

org/get-help/) offers an array of resources to help you determine whether you have an eating disorder and where you can find help.

It's important to learn to accept your body. Real bodies come in all shapes and sizes, and rarely correspond to the impossible fantasy bodies that turn up on TikTok and adorn fashion magazines. That doesn't mean that we shouldn't work on looking as great as possible (workouts in the gym are fine), but we shouldn't do it by not eating. Teenage brains and bodies are still developing and need proper nutrition.

Staying hydrated—Water helps your body regulate temperature, lubricate joints, recover from injury, and remove waste. It helps bring nutrients to our cells. It also helps produce bodily fluids like saliva and tears, and it protects your organs and tissues. When you're sick, hydration helps your skin and mucous membranes act as a barrier to bacteria that might enter the body (Remember when you had the flu? The doctor kept saying "Drink plenty of fluids!").

Most dermatologists will tell you that adequate hydration is one factor in maintaining healthy skin, nails, and hair.

Dehydration can lead to mood swings, difficulty concentrating, and cognitive impairment. It can also lead to urinary tract infections and heat strokes. When you're on a hike or out for a run, or when the temperature starts to creep up, be sure to carry a water bottle.

The amount of water that you need each day will obviously vary with your size and activity level (if you are training for a marathon, you'll need more than if you're on the sidelines cheering). Here are some tips for staying hydrated:

- Drink water consistently throughout the day, starting before breakfast.
- Drink while exercising—at least a glass before you start, and then at least that much every twenty to thirty minutes (if you're out in the sun, you'll need even more).
- Carry a reusable water bottle—it will remind you to keep drinking.
- Eat hydrating foods like watermelon, strawberries, and cantaloupe.
- Track your water consumption each day, to make sure that you drink enough.
- Remember, even if your brain isn't screaming "Thirsty, thirsty!" you still need to meet your requirement.
- You can substitute flavored water if you wish, but avoid those that will add calories to your diet.
- Tea and unsweetened juice are also good alternatives to water, though coffee is a diuretic and can be dehydrating.

We tend to take water for granted, but it's basic to our survival. So, drink enough. If your urine is darker than usual, your body probably needs more liquid.

Learn to cook—The best way to ensure that you're eating healthy is to cook the food you eat. That way, you know what goes into it, and you can control the portions. See the Further Reading section below for some cookbooks to help you get started.

Try cooking with your friends, rotating whose house will host weekly or monthly dinners (or lunches or brunches on weekends). Cooking should not be not intimidating.

Takeaways—Healthy eating can become a habit that lasts throughout your life. It's not hard to develop good eating habits once you're armed with information about the available choices. Investigate. Read the labels on foods. Develop strategies that help you avoid peer pressure. It's science, but it's also common sense. Of course, if you need help figuring out the right choices, get help from someone you trust. *Right now, you are eating for the rest of your life.*

Questions to ask yourself and to discuss:

- Have I tried to develop good eating habits, so that I naturally choose nutrient-dense foods?
- Do I read food labels to help me determine whether a food is nutrient-dense?
- Do I limit my consumption of salt, refined sugar, and fats that are unhealthy?
- Do I get enough fiber? Do I know how to identify foods that are high in fiber when there is no nutritional label?
- Do I drink more coffee than I should? Do I avoid energy drinks with excessive levels of caffeine?
- Do I think about the possible long-term effects of the foods that I choose?

Further reading

McManus, Katherine E. "10 superfoods to boost a healthy diet." Harvard Medical School, October 3, 2022. https://www.health.harvard.edu/blog/10-superfoods-to-boost-a-healthy-diet-2018082914463.

Lond-Caulk, Tina. *Eat Well and Feel Great: The Teenager's Guide to Nutrition and Health.* Green Tree, 2023.

Michaud, Noah. *The Healthy Cookbook for Teens: 100 Fast and Easy Delicious Recipes.* Callisto Teens, 2019.

Naidoo, Uma. *The Food Mood Connection.* Short Books, 2020.

van Tulleken, Chris. *Ultra-Processed People: The Science Behind Food that Isn't Food.* W. W. Norton, 2023.

USDA. *Dietary Guidelines for Americans 2020–2025.* https://www.dietaryguidelines.gov/sites/default/files/2021-03/Dietary_Guidelines_for_Americans-2020-2025.pdf.

Chapter III

Healthy habits strengthen you

The habits that you develop now—as a teenager—could determine how you live as an adult. This is because habits tend to stay with us. This chapter about healthy habits is about setting yourself up, right now, to be the best version of yourself in the future. It treats habits as a major element in your development. With the right habits, you'll develop in the right way, assuming that nothing deters you (a possibility that this and later chapters will consider).

What are habits? A habit is a behavior that is performed consistently. It can be physical, such as combing your hair every morning, or mental, such as preparing a checklist to ensure you're prepared for the day. Good habits are skills. They can be learned through repetition and a willingness to get past obstacles associated with their formation and continuation. Consider Dr. Atul Gawande's *A Checklist Manifesto: How to Get Things Right*, showing how surgeons use checklists routinely—that is, habitually—to ensure that they miss nothing during a long, tiring operation where they are responsible for teams of doctors, nurses, and assistants. Gawande demonstrates how developing and then following the right habits makes his job more straightforward and saves patients' lives.

Humans are creatures of habit. We form habits through conditioning—we do something again and again until the action comes naturally. By creating good habits now—managing your time, taking exercise breaks—you contribute to your overall health without having to stop, think, and remember to do what's best for you. You enhance your resilience by being *prepared* to act quickly and beneficially.

The US government's Occupational Safety and Health Administration (OSHA) requires that firefighters complete annual refresher courses to maintain their skills in key areas such as emergency response and the handling of hazardous materials. We cite this directive in the Further Reading section. OSHA wants these skills to become habits, so that if a firefighter is called on, say, to handle hazardous materials, they won't have to stop, consult a manual, try to remember what they learned during his training, and only then take action. Precious minutes could be lost if they don't act spontaneously.

Likewise, the prominent news site FireRescue1 states: "It's helpful to develop a tool training schedule to ensure members' skills remain automatic." It goes on to explain what this entails, which, applied generally, should be a mantra when we think about good habits:

> Too often, we train our members on a tactic or tool until they can simply perform the task. Ideally, we should drill

on it enough until we can't screw it up. This level of competency is essential to perform under stress. So, train and then revisit the training to make sure the skills are cemented and becoming automatic.

The formation of good habits is a serious, life-enhancing, life-*saving* practice. In fact, you could extrapolate from firefighters to nurses, teachers, dentists—anyone who must size up a situation and act quickly and proficiently. People with responsibility, to themselves or others, should not have to reinvent the wheel. While you're not an emergency responder, you still need to perform up to your highest potential, without always starting from square one ("Do I need to get enough sleep before this exam?"). That's where habits come in. You do what you need to do, without rethinking.

That's not to say that you shouldn't modify a habit, adapting it to changing circumstances or to some new, pivotal knowledge. Think of the firefighter, on the job for twenty years while technology keeps changing. Their habits evolve accordingly. They've made a habit of developing the right habits, always keeping up to date. They've also retained certain bedrock habits like paying attention to detail which, in the case of the new high-rise manual, allows their habits to change. The point is that, while habits don't preclude the exercise of judgment, they're nonetheless stabilizing. They help us get through the day and respond—not just to the big challenges, but to all the little forks in the road where we could respond one way but it's better to do something else.

The importance of Now. Humans routinely make excuses for bad habits ("It's okay not to wear a helmet if I'm biking in the park—there aren't any cars!"). We rationalize our lack of motivation for changing them ("Everybody has a joint on weekends—there's no school, so I don't need to be sharp"). Our brains are wired to make us feel better by telling ourselves little lies. Yet making excuses for bad habits is itself a bad habit. It interferes with developing good habits, creating a kind of cognitive dissonance where we know what we should do, but avoid the hard work of doing it now. In *Laws of Human Behavior: Steps Toward Hard Science*, Donald Pfaff and Sandra Sherman provide an example of such cognitive gymnastics, based on how smokers maneuver around the obvious need to quit.

> [A] smoker may admit that his habit causes cancer but, since he's addicted, he cannot imagine quitting. So, how does he "function"? He convinces himself that while the research is right, it applies only to the general population—special people, like him, are too tough to be bothered by a few mutant cells. Thus, he keeps on smoking, maybe even telling himself that it makes him even stronger ("Hey, didn't tough guys like Bogart smoke?"). Notice that in order to cope with all the adverse publicity and insistent warning labels, the smoker can both minimize the risk and attribute actual benefits to his habit. This way, he keeps on smoking—stress-free. The smoker might also have justified his behavior by citing worse alternatives, for example, claiming that his favorite brands are kinder, gentler versions of their French and Turkish counterparts ("A few Gauloises and you're dead!"). After a while, he might just tune out any

information that continues to challenge his rationalizations ("I've heard it all before, and I'm still here").

Notice how the smoker in this example engages in infinite postponement. He keeps thinking up ways to defer his better judgment, even while he *knows* the reasons to break his habit and take corrective action. Habits exert a powerful pull on our psyches and intellects. We go to great lengths—tying ourselves into mental knots—to avoid changing them. This chapter will discuss ways to break bad habits. But first, consider your own current take on habits.

We should accept the importance of *now* in terms of acknowledging our excuses—that is, being honest with ourselves—and developing a foundation of good habits as our brains and bodies develop. Some habits will be immediately useful, like leaving enough time to study for exams. Others will last a lifetime, like getting enough sleep. We will also develop new habits as our circumstances change. But the point is not to procrastinate in forming good habits now, especially those that are immediately useful to making the most of our lives. Good habits are the infrastructure of our physical, mental, and psychological well-being.

Good habits. Here are some habits that you can cultivate now. We've chosen sixteen, but based on your own needs, you can swap in others. Of course, any list this long may seem daunting. But good habits must start somewhere. You might choose a few that seem immediately relevant to your personal circumstances ("I know I grab Pop Tarts every morning, when I should eat a heathy breakfast"), and then move on to a few more. At the bottom of this list, we offer tips on how to develop a habit and make it stick. One tip is not to make it a lonely pursuit, which puts all the burden on you. When you've chosen a few habits to start with, ask your friends or family members for support as you work through to the next set.

- Eat a healthy, well-balanced diet, based on the USDA *Guidelines* discussed in Chapter II.
- Get enough sleep—teenagers need eight to ten hours per night, so arrange your life to get the sleep you need.
- Allow enough time to study so that you don't have to cram before exams.
- Begin writing papers far enough in advance so that you can review your work after a day or two—one rule of good writing is that it always takes longer than you think it will.
- Take frequent exercise breaks—your head will be clearer when you return to your work, and you will also feel less stiff.
- Keep physically active—find an activity you enjoy, and then do it. Just plain walking is great exercise.
- Use your exercise breaks to think about what you're working on—you'll be amazed at how creative you can be when you're not directly focused.
- Manage your time effectively—make checklists, establish priorities, acknowledge how long things will *really* take, don't allow yourself to be distracted online.

- Act deliberately—slow down and consider your options. Don't act impetuously, since some mistakes are hard to correct.
- Share your concerns—don't keep your anxieties bottled up. If you need professional help, then get it.
- Socialize with people who share your values, and who won't pressure you into behaviors that you know can be harmful.
- Practice continuous learning—read books outside your class assignments; follow the news so that you're well informed; pursue a hobby (like chess) where you have the chance to perfect your skills.
- Develop financial literacy—ask your parents, or someone you trust, about how to save and grow your money, how to take prudent financial risks, and how to plan for your financial future.
- Practice intellectual independence—rather than asking how something should be, figure it out for yourself by reading, talking with others, debating.
- Listen while you're talking with people—don't just keep thinking of the next thing to say. People notice and will resent it.
- When bad stuff happens, allow yourself to grieve, then pick yourself up and keep going—if you made a mistake, acknowledge it, fix it, learn from it, and try to do better next time.

In addition, we've generalized these habits into three overarching practices, which we call "good orientations." We'll discuss these in more detail just because they call for a significant mental commitment.

- Cultivate resilience—be open to changing circumstances and life's surprises. Bitterness and anger are pointless. Regret consumes a lot of energy. Stay positive, creative, and engaged in what's happening.
- Set realistic goals so that you do not disappoint yourself—we'll say more about this because it's complicated, but for now, practice being yourself without trying to be someone else who seems awesome but isn't *you*.
- Practice mindfulness—be aware of yourself in the moment.

All of these can make you happier (as in acing an exam). They can make you feel like a responsible person, actively in charge of your life. Remember that while some habits just sneak up on us, most result from an initial choice ("I want to eat a healthy breakfast," "I want to set realistic goals"). Of course, it may be easier to develop some habits ("If my mom stops buying Pop Tarts, I'll *have* to eat something else") than to struggle with developing others ("I *must* listen when people talk"). There is no harm in starting with the less challenging. Once you get into the habit of forming good habits, and become comfortable following the tips (see below) that can help you form them, you can tackle those that seem more difficult.

There are well-defined pathways to developing a good habit. In the following example, a teen sets out to *replace* a bad habit with a better one, which is harder than just starting a new one (where there is no previous baggage). But in this case, it's still not *that* hard because the new habit can be developed with relatively modest behavioral changes. We've designed this example in terms of development/replacement because, in most cases, this bivalent process reflects what actually occurs when we're trying to form new habits. If you are only concerned with forming a new habit, and not also with replacing a bad one (or at least some practice that's suboptimal), then you can modify these steps accordingly.

Here's what to do:

Set a goal—Clearly define the habit you want to develop ("I want to eat a healthier breakfast that no longer includes Pop Tarts and other sugary packaged foods").

Create reinforcing conditions—Eliminate temptations as much as possible. If your goal is to stop eating Pop Tarts, then make sure they're not within reach. You should just eat something else until you get used to it (and like it!).

Devise a plan—Create a detailed plan, using cues to help you remember ("When I'm in a rush for school, that's my cue to pop some whole wheat bread in the toaster—it'll be hot like a Pop Tart, but it won't *be* a Pop Tart"). Notice how this plan takes advantage of similarity (something hot from the toaster) to design a more congenial replacement. A good plan should be psychologically effective and build tangible satisfaction (something hot!) into the new habit. Satisfaction does not come just from feeling virtuous.

Another way of viewing this Pop Tart-for-toast trade is that it interrupts the cycle of cues that reinforce the bad habit. Thus, it interrupts the current cue/routine/reward cycle by finding a different reward—you're replacing the Pop Tart with something else that still tastes good but is better for you.

Make satisfaction apparent from the start—Find ways to make repeating the habit enjoyable from the outset ("I'll vary what I spread on my toast—one day peanut butter, another day hummus, then maybe mashed avocado"). Notice the variety, even though the toast—the Pop Tart replacement—remains the same. The point is to sustain your level of satisfaction so that you don't lose interest after a few tries.

Start small—Initiate changes without triggering your brain's fight-or-flight mechanism. Maybe top your toast with a small amount of *something* sweet, then over a few weeks reduce the amount until you don't miss the sweetness at all. Peanut butter still tastes great even without jelly.

Use reminders—Leave notes for yourself where the bad habit occurs (in this case, the kitchen) to help you rethink the bad habit before you're tempted. Be bold! For example, "Do you really want to consume 120 empty calories?" "Do you like being a junk food addict?"

Change your environment—Identify where you are at greatest risk. Since this bad habit occurs near the fridge, try to avoid it. You can put the bread and the toaster in another part of the kitchen, and keep an avocado nearby.

Be flexible—Allow for some flexibility in your plan. If your family has run out of whole wheat bread, try toasted pita or even an English muffin. You don't want to get derailed just because your usual MO needs some adjustment. You might even *choose* to adjust it, so long as you're still not reverting to the old habit (Pop Tarts).

Get support—Find people who can support you as you develop your new habit ("I'll ask my sister to have breakfast with me—she's into health, and will totally get what I'm trying to do"). It's important to seek support from people who are not just sympathetic, but on board with what you're trying to do; understand your motivations; and may even join what you're doing (if they haven't already adopted similar practices). If they've been through challenges like yours, that's even better.

Reward yourself—Anticipating a reward can motivate you to keep on toward your goal ("If I can go two weeks without a Pop Tart, I'll get that new retro T-shirt I've wanted"). You can set up a system of rewards, so that with every milestone—maybe *every* two weeks—you're entitled to a reward.

Track your progress—Use an app or other method to track your progress, and to remind you if you need reminding. Just seeing all the days without Pop Tarts line up, one after another, is encouraging. It stiffens your resolve. It's ego-boosting, so make your ego *depend*, in part, on not eating Pop Tarts. Here's an analogy: If you run, isn't it great to see all the miles go by on your smartwatch?

Keeping track is also a venerable strategy. In the eighteenth century, before there was any technology other than pen and paper for tracking one's progress, Benjamin Franklin's *Autobiography* was a record of how he dealt with (or failed to deal with) temptation.

Be patient—If you experience slip-ups, learn from them, and don't be discouraged. Remind yourself that your goal is worth the effort. Most importantly, don't be angry with yourself if your progress seems less than linear, provided you're really trying.

Don't play mind games with yourself—The smoker in the example above always had some rationale for not quitting ("Hey, didn't tough guys like Bogart smoke?"). But if you don't meet your goal, don't play mind games to justify falling short. Just be patient; call on your support team; anticipate the next reward if you can make it to the next milestone.

Adopting good habits takes work, especially if the new ones are supposed to replace older ones. But adopting good habits is a skill. You learn the skill—for example, by following the tips outlined above—so that adopting subsequent habits is easier. You have a skill that, in effect, becomes a habit ("I've developed the habit of forming better habits"). The trick to habit formation is to stick with it.

Good orientations. The first sixteen habits listed above are self-explanatory—for example, staying active—and some, at least, are easy to figure out based on your experience or discussions elsewhere in this *Guide*. However, the last three practices on the list (which, as we said, "call for a significant mental commitment") may be open to various interpretations. What is resilience, and how does it become a habit? What does it mean to set realistic goals? What is mindfulness in the context of teenage health and wellness? In what follows, we try to answer these questions.

Resilience—Resilience is the capacity to bounce back from adversity. You remain positive, engaged, ready for the next opportunity. Your energy isn't consumed by anger or regret. If you get bent out of shape, you don't break, and finally you find yourself—again—in a healthy place.

Consider an analogy from materials science (which studies how metals, meshes, and ceramics resist fracturing under stress):

When a sufficient load is applied to metal or other structural, it will cause the material to change shape. The change in shape is called deformation. A temporary shape change that is self-reversing after the force is removed, so that the object returns to its original shape, is called elastic deformation. In other words, elastic deformation is a change in shape of a material at low stress that is recoverable after the stress is removed . . .

When the stress is sufficient to permanently deform the metal, it is called plastic deformation.

This passage, from the Center for Nondestructive Evaluation, Iowa State University, cited in the Further Reading section, explains how some materials—like those used in airplanes—may experience stress but won't collapse. Their shape is "recoverable." They'll *resume* their functionality.

Of course, you're not some aluminum alloy in an airplane wing. But you do experience stress, and you *can* bounce back. In fact, unlike metal, you can bounce back better, having learned from the experience and incorporated what you've learned into a new MO ("I was so depressed after I got a C in algebra—but now I'm taking AP math because I learned to buckle down and study!"). You just need to be prepared for the next hard knock and recognize that you're able to get past it. In other words, you need to get into the habit of being resilient—or, rather, you need to develop the traits that, together, can make you naturally resilient.

But how?

In "Building Your Resilience," the American Psychological Association suggests practices that, in some personal combination, can help us bounce back from trauma.

- Make connections with people and build strong relationships with family and friends.
- Avoid seeing crises as insurmountable problems.
- Accept that change is part of living, and there are circumstances you cannot alter.
- Move toward your goals, but make them realistic.
- Take decisive actions, and act on adverse situations as much as you can rather than being passive.
- Look for opportunities to discover more about yourself and gain an increased sense of self-worth.
- Nurture a confident, positive view of yourself.
- Keep events in perspective, and do not blow them out of proportion.
- Maintain a hopeful outlook, and visualize what you want.
- Take care of yourself by paying attention to your emotional and physical needs.[1]

In many ways, this *Guide* is an extension of these points. It urges you to set realistic goals, and to consider your emotional

---

1 www.apa.org/topics/resilience

and physical well-being. It focuses on building relationships—both the strategic kind, that will help you through a crisis, and those that will last forever. What's important about resilience is that as a teenager, your life is just beginning. You can't allow yourself to get bogged down in disappointment ("How will I get into an Ivy if I didn't ace the PSAT?"). You figure out possible work-arounds ("Hey, there are dozens of great schools I can get into"). You learn from the experience, try harder, and maybe surprise yourself on the SAT with some impressive results. The point is to keep going, and not to give up.

If you practice the traits listed above, you'll begin to be habitually resilient. You'll notice the change. Resilience creates a feedback loop where, once you begin to be resilient in some areas, you'll find that you're also resilient in others. You can start now by taking an inventory of your resilience-producing traits—Do I maintain a hopeful outlook? Am I paying attention to my physical and emotional needs? If you find you're deficient in some areas, work on them. Of course, while you may not adopt all the recommended traits, we can't think of one that you wouldn't want to.

Setting realistic goals—As noted above, setting realistic goals is a good habit. It's part of becoming resilient. But goal-setting is tricky. We want to be the best we can be, and don't want to disappoint ourselves by setting goals that are too high or otherwise inconsistent with our sense of ourselves. We should make it a habit to think about who we are; to recognize our skills, interests, and personality; and then be *that person*—nobody else—as effectively as possible. If you'd love to be a quantative analyst and start a hedge fund, but your math skills are subpar, then don't spin your wheels. Don't feel like you've lost out. Instead, try to determine who *you* are and what *you* can be. This entails reflection and honest self-assessment (another important habit), which we discuss in Chapter IV. You should talk with a guidance counselor about which goals are realistic based on all the factors that go into such a decision. Then you can develop the right habits to help you work toward them (e.g., studying hard, continuous learning) and help you succeed at them.

You're not giving up a dream. You're not closing off options (you can always change plans if your circumstances alter). But you *are* saving yourself disappointment. It's been shown that once people give up an unrealistic goal for one that's appropriate, they end up being happy with their choice.

Also, you're not accepting a dumbed-down future. You're going in a different direction. As MacArthur Prize–winner Howard Gardner showed in *Frames of Mind: The Theory of Multiple Intelligences*, "intelligence" is not limited to verbal and logical/mathematical skills as measured on standard IQ tests. It can be artistic, musical, kinesthetic (related to movement, like dance), and even social, introspective, or grounded in environmental awareness. Setting realistic goals can be a wide-open process, based on self-discovery. You just need to develop habits, like self-reflection, that will help you set them.

In every case, your habits should be aligned with working toward your goals. If you plan to be a dancer, you should practice for hours and hours every day. If you *do* think you can be a quantative analyst, then make mathematics a priority—get into the habit of understanding the underlying concepts, rather than just solving problems by rote application of a formula.

Don't just assume that you have a "natural" talent that doesn't need to become a skill. Everything goal-related is harder than it seems, so commit to working at it.

Mindfulness—We hear this term a lot. It has various meanings in popular culture—especially among celebrity influencers. But what this *Guide* means by it is this: paying attention in the present moment (the moral equivalent of not crossing the street with your head in your phone). You immerse yourself in your thoughts, emotions, sensations. You examine them and bring them to the surface ("Hey, I never realized I like rainy days—they make me feel calm, like nature still has a chance"). You get in touch with yourself. When practiced regularly, mindfulness enhances our understanding of how we perceive things and process our perceptions. It helps to relieve stress. It can be a springboard to creativity.

Mindfulness may be the ultimate habit to cultivate. It should be integral to how we proceed through the world. But it's so easy to miss with all the multitasking we are called on to perform, and the information overload that seems like our natural (and eternal) state. We are afraid of missing out. Our brains have a mechanism (selective perception) to help screen out all this activity so that we can slow down and be receptive to our surroundings. As Donald Pfaff and Sandra Sherman observe in *Laws of Human Behavior*:

New York City is a cacophony of sounds: police sirens, ambulances, high-rise construction, motorcycles, eighteen-wheelers, all-night sidewalk cafés, drive-by DJs. Yet somehow, pedestrians hear the birds, and birdwatchers identify their distinct calls. How? Humans regularly deploy "selective perception," filtering out sensory stimuli that are undesirable or irrelevant so that what remains can be processed into coherent, desirable sounds and images.

In a manner of speaking, we can learn to hear what we want to hear and can see what we want to see. It is a type of cognitive bias that can become unconscious.

Part of being mindful is permitting our capacity for selective perception to allow us to focus, to tune out all the noise so that we can look inward. We should allow ourselves some time every day to pay attention to our thoughts.

There are also several practical ways to support our attempts to be mindful. One of the best is to detach from our devices for a while, and be alone in our own heads. As Donald Pfaff demonstrates in *Origins of Human Socialization*, neuroscience is now concerned that our brains cannot process all the multidimensional noise of the digital world. They evolved to perform optimally in much smaller social units, even though—currently—technology is making all of us simultaneously present to all of us. So perhaps, even just sometimes, we are better off without it. At the very least, we owe it to ourselves to eliminate distractions, which is the first step toward becoming mindful.

Help with bad habits. If you have developed a bad habit—for example, smoking—now is the time to break it. As illustrated above, you can replace bad habits ("I hate exercise for its own sake!") with good ones ("I'll just take a walk—I know it's good for me"). Breaking bad habits and replacing them with good ones are usually part of a multidimensional, continuous process. You work on both simultaneously. If you need professional help, perhaps with binge eating, then now is the time to get it.

Habits are just not physical; they can be intellectual ("Algebra is boring, so I'll skip those demonstration problems") and even psychological ("For some reason, I just act impetuously"). It's therefore necessary to ask, "What are my good habits? My bad ones? How can I improve?" Keep the good ones, and work on shaking the others. Don't feel guilty about your habits. Rather, find support and work at finding better ones.

Takeaways—Habits are like roadmaps into the future. If we develop good habits, they'll lead us to a future we'd like to live in. Bad habits, however, are extremely hard to break and can lead toward a less pleasant future. So, it's important to develop good habits now. If we need help discarding bad habits, we should seek it. Along the way, we should practice mindfulness and pay attention to what we're thinking. We can't ever treat our mind's processes casually.

Questions to ask yourself and to discuss:

- What habits should I try to develop now? Which ones should I try to ditch?
- Do I take seriously the idea that forming good habits now will be useful later?
- Do I have sources of support as I work on my habits?

- If I am having trouble replacing a bad habit with a good one, am I willing to seek appropriate help?
- Do I practice mindfulness?
- Am I working toward becoming resilient?

Further reading

Beck, Andrew. "How often should firefighters train on—not just *with*—their tools and equipment?" FireRescue1, November, 13, 2023. https://www.firerescue1.com/making-the-cut-the-definitive-guide-to-firefighting-tools/how-often-should-firefighters-train-on-not-just-with-their-tools-and-equipment.

Franklin, Benjamin. *Autobiography*. 1771. W.W. Norton & Co., 1986.

Gardner, Howard. *Frames of Mind: The Theory of Multiple Intelligences*. Basic Books, 1983. Note: this is the classic text. Dr. Gardner has since written several follow-up books on multiple intelligences.

Gawande, Atul. *The Checklist Manifesto: How to Get Things Right*. Metropolitan Books, 2010.

Iowa State University. "Elastic/Plastic Deformation." https://www.nde-ed.org/Physics/Materials/Structure/deformation.xhtml.

Kabat-Zinn, Jon. *Mindfulness for Beginners*. Sounds True, 2016.

OSHA. "Firefighter Annual Refresher Training Guidance." https://www.dhses.ny.gov/system/files/documents/2021/12/fire-dept-annual-refresher.pdf.

Pfaff, Donald, and Sandra Sherman. *Laws of Human Behavior: Steps Toward Hard Science*. MIT Press, 2025.

Pfaff, Donald. *Origins of Human Socialization*. Academic Press, 2021.

Southwick, Steven, and Dennis Charney. *Resilience: The Science of Mastering Life's Greatest Challenges*. Cambridge University Press, 2018.

Wood, Wendy. *Good Habits, Bad Habits: The Science of Making Positive Changes That Stick*. Farrar, Straus and Giroux, 2019.

Chapter IV

Self-reflection helps you find your way

During the first half of the twentieth century, the poet T. S. Eliot published *Four Quartets*, one of whose poems included "Burnt Norton," with lines that imagine a "still point . . . where past and future are gathered." This state is such a paradox (how can what-was and what-will-be be simultaneous?) that it must exist separately, outside daily existence. Of course, past and future can only fuse together in the mind, into a version of time that makes no distinction between them. We're outside the sort of time that we usually inhabit, which we measure in tiny segments. Here, everything flows. It's a type of Now that is a series of Nows. The idea is a good introduction to the practice of self-reflection. It suggests that as we draw ourselves into our minds, slow down, and think, the activity is intense. What we've done and may yet do coalesce: "Who am I? Where am I going?" We focus on ourselves, and for a while, that's all that matters.

What is self-reflection?—The term "self-reflection" may have as many meanings as there are practitioners of it (from "I always contemplate why I'm here" to "Maybe I'll figure out how to get through the week"). In general, however, it involves a type of quiet meditation on your character, actions, and motives—the qualities of mind and heart that only you can discern, and that make you do what you do. The emphasis is on internality. You literally reflect, as a mirror would, on yourself.

The practice goes back a long way in the Western tradition. Consider the French philosopher, René Descartes (1596–1650), known for his famous statement "Cogito, ergo sum" (I think, therefore I am). Descartes's emphasis on the role of self-reflection, and of the thinking self in the process of philosophical inquiry, profoundly shaped how we *think* about thinking. So have the plays of William Shakespeare (1564–1616), who features interior monologues—the characters' introspections, which we overhear—in plays such as *Hamlet* and *Othello*.

More recently and closer to home, the American transcendentalist Henry David Thoreau published *Walden: or, Life in the Woods* (1854), which describes his experiences of living a life of solitude and self-reflection in the woods near Concord, Massachusetts. His work reflects upon reflecting, which, in a way, demonstrates what self-reflection is: free-form, free association, where one thought leads to another but may also double back on itself. There are no rules. You are inside your own head. But there is one major difference with what we call the unconscious. Self-reflection is entirely conscious. It's the product of intense self-awareness, such that Thoreau could record his reflections (including the process of how they unfolded) and publish them. *Walden* is now a classic of American literature.

In the spirit of Thoreau—though we don't suggest that you spend two years in the woods—the *Guide*, with its accompanying questions, is structured around encouraging you to think about yourself, and look inwards. "Am I working out too much, and endangering my health?" "Do I feel depressed and, if so, what may be causing it?" Looking inward is a prelude to course correction, if necessary. It's also a prelude to sharing how you feel and seeking advice. It's not just some lonely, self-involved pursuit for Hamlet and other tortured souls. It's an everyday practice for everyone. It's a way of helping you decide what's next.

Some people find that keeping a diary helps to crystallize their thoughts. Novels have been written in the form of a diary—for example, *Bridget Jones's Diary* by Helen Fielding—because novelists like to explore the mind's inner workings. You can find dozens if you search. Going back two hundred years, *Robinson Crusoe* (1719), one of the first proto-novels in English, situates Crusoe on a distant island where—compelled to reflect on his experiences—he keeps a diary. Daniel Defoe, *Crusoe's* author, was steeped in the Puritan tradition of diary-keeping, which held that if you keep a faithful record of what you did each day and your reflections on it, God would reveal his purpose for your life.

Self-reflection is woven into Western literature and philosophy because people have realized, from a variety of perspectives, that we need an inner life. We need to think quietly about ourselves. Maybe we'll discover that we owe someone an apology—or that they owe us one. Maybe we'll think about our summer weight loss, and how great it is to fit into those shorts lying at the bottom of the drawer. The point is that reflection helps us to maintain equilibrium and bring issues to the surface when it's finally time to think acknowledge them ("I couldn't think about those extra pounds all winter, but now I can!").

Self-refection does not just have to be about important personal questions, like where to go to college or whether to break up with someone you've been dating. Sometimes it's good to think about lesser concerns—you're still experiencing yourself *as* yourself, distinct from the crowd, unique. You can laugh at your own jokes. Who cares?

Finally, while self-reflection is a counterpart to mindfulness (see Chapter III), it's not the same. Self-reflection is less focused on the moment. It's potentially concerned with the grand sweep of your life. It's more utilitarian. Together with mindfulness, it helps you to cope—and maintain your mental health. It sets you up for the future because, unlike mindfulness, it helps to integrate how you feel now with how you may feel about some future version of yourself. The emphasis is on "may," since you don't have to make definitive decisions. You can keep coming back to questions from new perspectives, with new ideas. Self-reflection is a process where everything is negotiable—and you're on both sides of the negotiation. If your conclusions are provisional, that's still fine. There's always the next time. You go with the flow.

The benefits—We've already mentioned some of the benefits of self-reflection, but here we want to line them up with many more, so that when you reflect on yourself you can try for those that matter most to you.

- *Builds your self-concept.* Psychologists use the term "self-concept" to describe your beliefs about yourself—how you construct your identity. As applied to teenagers, the term is tricky. At this stage, you want to fit in with your peers, but you also want to distinguish yourself ("I'm not just a face in the crowd"). Self-reflection helps you build your self-concept, how you feel about yourself. Unless you know, how are you going to understand the identity that you want to project into the world?

- *Contributes to your self-development.* What are your strengths and weaknesses? How can you improve? Through self-reflection, you can reverse the cycle of repetition where you just keep doing what you've always done—perhaps hurting others, perhaps yourself. You begin to understand yourself and develop emotional intelligence.

- *Develops self-awareness.* Unlike self-concept, "self-awareness" applies to your current attitudes and dispositions. Let's take an example. Instead of acting impetuously, without regard for your motivations, through self-awareness you can confront your motivations and try to understand them ("I realize that I don't like careless dressers, so I often ignore their redeeming qualities"). You can better change what needs to be changed—if only so that you like yourself better.

- *Sharpens your communication skills.* If you understand what you feel, you can better express yourself. You can be more honest and straightforward.
- *Develops awareness of your core values.* What do you believe about the world and your place in it? What role do your values play in your life? ("I plan to volunteer for ROTC in college, because saving democracy really matters to me"). Through self-reflection, you can ensure that your actions and your values are consistent, that you don't just do something because everyone else is doing it. You are your own person. Chapter V will discuss core values in detail.
- *Helps in evaluating your options.* As we get older, our range of options becomes narrower, more constricted. But right now, with so few obligations (apart from going to school and doing well), your range of options is vast. "What interests do I want to cultivate?" "How can I make a difference in my community?" Self-reflection helps you to evaluate your options by foregrounding your core values and what you believe are your abilities.
- *Makes you accountable to yourself.* In the privacy of your own mind, you can hold yourself accountable without telling anyone else. ("Okay, I grabbed a jar of cinnamon at the supermarket because the line was so long—it was shoplifting, and I'm ashamed of myself".) Self-reflection helps you process shame and move on. It helps you confront your flaws and

impulses, which you might be less inclined to do out in the open.

- *Promotes meta-cognition.* In other words, it helps you think about your thought processes. Do you like to skip over details and focus on the big picture? Will this trait serve you well if you want to be a lawyer, a scientist, or a journalist? If you tend toward confirmation bias (selecting among facts based on those that suit you) will this hinder your self-presentation as fair and equitable? Thinking about how you think, especially in the context of fraught situations, will help you navigate the world with honesty and integrity.

- *Helps in stress management.* You can sort out the various stressors in your life and think about how to deal with them. In Chapter I, we discuss stress management, in which self-reflection is a key element.

- *Assists in long- and short-term planning.* You have lots to do (writing papers, taking exams, buying your mother a birthday present). How do you organize all this stuff which, right now, is stressing you out? How do you keep from resenting your obligations, when they are just part of living a full life? Self-reflection is a form of personal logistics. It helps you establish your priorities. It helps you plan and make changes to your plans. If you know where you are going—rather than just flailing around—you feel less stressed.

Picture this scenario. You're deciding which colleges to apply to, and the array of choices is vast.

What do you do? You ask yourself questions about the sort of person you are and what matters to you in an education. "Am I the artsy type, or would I like a geekier school? Would I like a school in an urban setting, so that I can develop my interest in urban ecology, or would I prefer a more rural school where I can paint wildlife in its natural habitat?" Once you know yourself better, your planning will be easier.

- *Improves your relationships.* If you understand yourself and are better able to communicate your feelings to others, you will be further along in establishing and maintaining strong relationships. You'll understand what you want from a relationship, and you'll be more empathetic. Recognizing your own humanity—including all your faults—is the first step toward recognizing and accepting others' humanity.

- *Improves your resilience.* Resilience is the capacity to bounce back from adversity. Self-reflection promotes resilience because, as we examine our motives and the reason(s) that we suffered the setback, we can equip ourselves so that we don't stay in the same place, spinning our wheels. Even if the setback is not our fault (a tornado, a drunk driver), we can reflect on avoidance mechanisms (build a tornado shelter, give erratic drivers a wide berth). Where it is our fault, we can think about ways to recover—even while not continuing in behaviors that will prolong the setback.

- *Helps with brain development and impulse control.* Hard thinking of any sort helps your brain develop.

Additionally, as you develop more brain pathways—and actually think through your decisions—you'll be less likely to act on impulse.

Self-reflection is a complex process. You can make it what you need it to be at any time, in any context. It doesn't have to be systematic ("First I will think about my communication skills, then about my values"). It doesn't have to be comprehensive, but through time, it can—in all its many facets—help strengthen you and define your individuality. It's another skill that, if practiced, can become a habit.

How can I become self-reflective? There are many ways to become self-reflective. In general, they represent personal choices: "What works for me? Am I more comfortable writing about my feelings, or just thinking quietly?" Whichever method you choose, you should eliminate distractions—no TV in the background, phones turned off. Just concentrate on yourself. Also, it's important to recognize that you're not obliged to resolve anything. You might reflect on the same question for weeks without reaching that "Aha!" moment. It's okay. The point is to honestly explore your thoughts (no mind games, no excuses). Remember, no one else is listening. But you are responsible to yourself, so take the effort seriously.

It's important to make self-reflection a habit. Once you begin, the practice will come naturally ("I actually *need* to find out what's in my head—I don't like this vague unease that keeps nagging me"). You'll find the time because, like all good habits, the practice will provide satisfaction. If you're worried about being self-involved, don't be. We need to get a firm purchase on ourselves before we can establish good relationships. Also, don't fail to reflect on yourself out of some mistaken notion that you're ordinary and boring ("I'm just like everyone else with typical teenage issues—who cares?"). You matter to yourself and, once you start to reflect on yourself, you'll probably discover that you're more interesting than you imagined. In this way, self-reflection is a good way to develop self-esteem.

Finally, you might ask, "What am I supposed to reflect on?" You can think about an experience, like missing a toss in a baseball game and why that may have happened ("Was I paying insufficient attention?" "Was I tired, and maybe shouldn't have played that day?"). Reflecting on an experience puts it into perspective. You can determine what role *you* played in how things turned out. You can better understand your interactions with others. But you don't have to reflect on anything so concrete as an experience—a missed toss, or even a missed bus ("Why am I chronically late?"). You can think about feelings that may be harder to situate and define. You can think about your goals ("Should I attend a big state university, or a small private college?") and how you're trying to accomplish them. You can think about the environment ("What can I do to help?" "How can I convince people to compost to reduce the amount of trash?"). Self-reflection can encompass anything that matters to you in the moment that you set out to reflect. Maybe it's just some upcoming exam. Let your thoughts be your guide.

If your thoughts drift toward the past ("How could we ever have broken up—we were so great together"), that's okay. While you shouldn't dwell on your regrets, the past still has stuff to teach you about yourself and your place in the world. It's an indelible part of your life, and sometimes you won't come to terms with it for years ("I finally figured out why I didn't get along with my brother!"). It's been said that the past is a foreign country. If you visit it, you can discover things.

Of course, if any of your thoughts are really disturbing, or maybe just reveal something about yourself that you don't know how to deal with, then you should seek help. You can talk to someone you trust and, maybe, a professional. Self-reflection can sometimes lead in unexpected directions. That's no reason to be afraid of it—it's necessary for your well-being—but you should deal with what you learn appropriately. There is a difference between allowing an issue to remain unresolved and letting it fester when what you need is help. You can make that decision on your own, or by sharing your concerns.

Here are some ways to start being self-reflective, though you can always practice more than one.

- *Keep a journal.* The value of journal-keeping is that when we write, we tend to be more careful and precise. We try to choose the correct word before committing it to some permanent record—for example, rather than saying "I felt unhappy" (which begs the question of *why*) we might say "I felt aggrieved" (which explains that you were hurt because you were treated unfairly). When you go back over your journal entries, which you should on a regular basis, they will cohere into a narrative that you can reflect on from a distance. You'll be able to trace your progress ("I guess I got over it, but it took a while"), and spot specific issues in your life that still need work.

Of course, it's important to keep your journal regularly—maybe set aside some time at the end of every day. It doesn't matter what medium you choose—if pen and paper feel quaint ("Hey, I'm not Thoreau"), then you can go digital. If you want to add illustrations ("That 200-year-old tree was a revelation!"), that's great. Ideally, your journal is an image of your thoughts. Don't feel obliged to share it with anyone. It's yours, and as private as your thoughts.

Journals are a form of self-discovery. Sometimes you don't know what you think until you require yourself to formulate sentences describing what you think. This type of self-discovery can be exciting. It can also provoke your creative impulses. Many short stories, and even novels, originated as a series of journal entries that outlined a compelling narrative. You may not *see* the story until you go back over what you've written, but then it may emerge. Of course, when you're writing on a day-to-day basis, you needn't think of yourself as writing a story with a plot, characters, and a distinct timeline. Just concentrate on what you need to externalize in the moment of your writing.

Finally, journal entries help you keep track of your progress as you face challenges ("I've now quit smoking for a week." "I've lost three pounds, and kept it off"). They can be a source of encouragement and keep you from berating yourself. If you need to work harder, they can help you formulate better plans ("Okay, I just have to eat breakfast, and not keep grabbing snacks until lunch"). Journaling has practical utility.

- *Stop and think when you can.* There are moments throughout the day when you can stop, think, and reflect. Maybe you're walking home from the bus stop. Maybe you're walking the dog or pulling weeds in your family's garden. To reflect, you don't have to be motionless or sitting in a chair. You just need to be sufficiently in your head so that whatever else you're doing isn't a distraction. Later, if you like, you can keep a more permanent record of what you thought about—you can think through your thoughts in spurts and *decide* what should go into your journal for more concentrated exploration. You might even make notes so you don't forget what you'd like to explore.

There's an old dictum that directs us to "improve the time." It means that we should enhance the quality of every moment and not let our time go to waste. There are interstitial moments in the day—moments between doing one thing and doing something else—that *can* be empty but don't need to be. Think of them as the temporal equivalent of empty calories which, instead, you can exchange for what's better for you. During these moments, you can reflect on yourself. You can deliberately make time for these moments or stretch them out a little. The point is to use them to reflect.

- *Meditate.* Meditation and mindfulness (discussed in Chapter III) are often equated. But they don't have to be. As a self-reflective practice, meditation has a useful objective—it's less thought for its own sake. You're trying to get hold of your life and make sense of its scattered pieces.

  During meditation, you can find a quiet spot, stop whatever you're doing, and just reflect. You don't need any special equipment, like a yoga mat, and you don't need to assume any special position. You just need to be still, so that you can reflect without being distracted. Your focus is inward.

  It's been observed that sometimes during meditation, our heart rate slows down, and we may breathe more slowly. This is an example of the mind/body connection discussed in Chapter I. We are engaged with our entire selves—which is entirely appropriate, since our focus *encompasses* our entire selves (our feelings, our experiences, what makes us *us*).

- *Have a conversation with yourself.* This may sound a little weird ("Don't schizophrenics talk to themselves?"), but it's actually helpful if you do it in the right spirit. Pose yourself a question—perhaps "How can I manage my time more effectively?"—and then literally try to articulate a cogent, even persuasive response. Talking out loud helps you find the right language. You can then interrogate that response by asking follow-up questions, until you've finally articulated a detailed, satisfying response that you can apply to your daily activities.

You'll notice that in conversation with yourself, you might start playing devil's advocate—"How can you say that!" "What about a totally different approach?" That's fine. Your brain is working. Self-criticism is crucial to honest self-reflection. It's a way of finally arriving at your own truth.

- *Talk with a friend, mentor, or even a therapist who understands you.* When we talk with people who care about and understand us, we often search our minds—our feelings—so that we can share our concerns with them. This process of turning inward so that we can finally externalize our concerns takes self-reflection to the next level. Such self-reflections occur in context of a relationship, even though we are the ultimate beneficiary.

Self-reflection is hard work, no matter the medium in which you pursue it. But the point is to keep at it. You may come back to the same questions again and again—each time, you're likely to approach them from different angles, with the benefit of what you've learned through previous reflection. Besides, there will always be new things to think about. Just make sure that self-reflection becomes a habit. Don't try to "protect" yourself from facing hard questions. Such questions can lead to important discoveries about yourself. In this sense, self-reflection is of great practical value. It's the opposite of self-indulgent. It's a necessary component of *leading* your life—that is, taking charge of it. You don't allow stuff to get away from you. Instead, you think about it, and incorporate it into how you *decide* to live.

Here is a case study of how self-reflection can be instrumental in untangling sensitive, difficult issues that only you can address. Of course, each person will have their own issues, but the process of honest, deeply personal reflection can help you arrive at an answer that is right for you.

Sexual orientation and gender identity—Sexuality is fundamental to human expression. You take it seriously. Though it just seems to happen ("I'm attracted to that person, and I barely know them"), it's actually a complex manifestation of the mind/body connection. While the urge seems physical, we process it in our heads. It has psychological implications. This means that ultimately, you should be comfortable in your body, which means that you should be psychologically comfortable with your sexual orientation and gender identity. You shouldn't have to spend endless time worrying about your sexuality. But to get to that point, you may have to spend considerable time figuring it out.

This is where self-reflection comes in.

Most people now recognize that sexuality is not just physically determined. That is, it's not just a question of whether you're stereotypically male or female based on the anatomical features you were born with. Because of the mind/body connection, we may find ourselves somewhere on a spectrum of sexual orientation (gay, lesbian, bisexual, etc.). We may discover our variant gender identity ("I was born a girl, but I feel like a boy"). The latter type of person is known as trans, for making a transition from one gender to another. The transition often goes beyond a mental one. Once they are sure of their trans identity, they may seek hormone therapy (male and female hormones can affect sexual characteristics, like growing breasts or sprouting a beard) or even surgery.

All people want to be comfortable in their bodies, *despite* anatomical features that may lead other people to impose their own expectations. In such cases, the mind (or rather the brain) overrules the body until they can be brought into sync. These people's feelings may be the product of personal history. They may reflect a fantasy of fluidity and liberation from social norms. No matter. It's *their* feelings, to which they are entitled. It's how they construct their identity so that they can be comfortable in their bodies (even if this causes some discomfort in the world at large).

This comfort, a type of equilibrium between the mind and body, doesn't always come easily.

If you are nonbinary or gender-nonconforming (that is, somewhere on the LGBTQ+ spectrum), you may struggle with *who you are*. But the first thing to understand is that there should be no shame in openly deciding—or, rather, discovering—who you are. It's not a decision so much as an awakening, a realization that you are who you are and it's okay. A healthy mind/body connection implies that you are finally comfortable in your sexuality. You may look for a supportive community. The point, however, is to be comfortable in yourself.

If you want to keep your self-discovery private, or maybe share it with only a few people, then that's your right. You can come out to people on your own terms, in your own time. The actor Richard Chamberlain, who played a hunk on television in the 1970s and '80s, didn't come out as gay until much later in life (he felt it would hurt his image, and hence his career, if he told anyone). Actor Rock Hudson never came out.

Of course, any reconsideration of your at-birth gender identity is a serious matter. It never hurts to talk with a professional counselor (who will always keep your confidences). Changing your gender identity is a huge, potentially irreversible undertaking—it can involve surgery and lifelong hormone therapy—so you really want to be sure before committing to it. Ask yourself: "Why do I feel the need to change?" "When did I start to feel this way?" "Am I responding to other people's influence, or is this my personal decision?" You don't need to rush into anything, but in the end, the decision is yours.

How can self-reflection specifically help teenagers? Apart from all the general benefits discussed above, self-reflection provides students with a way to evaluate their strengths and weaknesses and establish a path of positive self-evaluation that includes speaking to teachers and others about any negative issues. This helps students track their progress (or lack of it); analyze how and what they're learning; take ownership of their intellectual life; and ensure that their teachers understand their individual perception of disparities between how they're doing and how they think they should be doing. In other words, students can deploy self-reflection in practical ways that can promote their academic success.

Because self-reflection enhances self-awareness, teenagers can better recognize which of their personal characteristics they want to emphasize as they progress through school and professional life. For example, if they want to emphasize their artistic skills, even though they're demonstrably good in math, they can make those decisions early enough to affect their course of study. They'll be less likely to go in one direction because they're "supposed" to, only to realize later that they really had other skills they could have developed that could have suited them better professionally. So again, it's been shown that self-reflection can be a tool that teenagers can use to take ownership of their lives (including, in this case, their future).

It's important to begin now. You might say, "There's nothing complicated about me, so I can always practice self-reflection when I really have something to reflect on." But no matter how much is going on in your life—or whether you think nothing much is going on—you'd be wrong to dismiss your *need* to reflect on yourself. Ask yourself whether, perhaps, you just find the idea unappealing ("It's okay for mama's boys like Hamlet, but not me!"), or you're scared about what you may uncover. Ask yourself whether you just find it easier to spend an available half hour scrolling through TikTok. In effect, you should reflect on why you resist self-reflection. The fact is that everyone can benefit from it, especially because each person can make up their own rules.

While narcissism and self-absorption are unattractive traits, self-reflection is entirely different. Okay, you're turning inward for a while. But it's because you want to strengthen your relationships. It's because you want to manage your life successfully—in part, so that you're pulling your weight in society. Ultimately, self-reflection is a social practice. It helps you connect with people because you discover aspects of yourself that you can effectively share.

Try different approaches until you settle on one (or more) that work for you ("I'm comfortable keeping a journal—it's like a mini-vacation, and afterward I feel less stressed," "I like having short conversations with myself—it's like I'm in a play playing all the characters"). Self-reflection is one of those habits that grows on you, like taking a walk after the rain because everything smells so fresh. It's worth getting into now.

Takeaways—Self-reflection is a necessary part of growing into the person that we should be. It allows us to assimilate ideas about into some coherent version of ourselves. But we should always remain self-reflective, since those ideas can change with time. Self-reflection should become a habit. We should make time for it, no matter how busy we are. We should be willing to face hard questions about ourselves, and hold ourselves to account.

Questions to think about and discuss:

- Can I find a way to integrate self-reflection into my daily life?
- Am I willing to think about difficult, even painful questions?

- Will I try various means of self-reflection, and settle on one (or more) with which I'm comfortable?
- Do I feel accountable to myself, so that I don't play mind games when I reflect on myself?
- Am I able to eliminate distractions in my surroundings, so that my self-reflection is effective?

Further reading

Bloom, Harold. *Shakespeare: The Invention of the Human.* Riverhead Books, 1998.

Defoe, Daniel. *Robinson Crusoe.* Wordsworth Editions, 1719.

Eliot, T. S. *Complete Poems and Plays.* Faber and Faber, 1958. (See Section II of "Four Quartets" for cited language.)

Fielding, Helen. *Bridget Jones's Diary.* Penguin, 1996.

Shakespeare, William. *Hamlet* (1604/05) and *Othello* (1603).

Thoreau, Henry David. *Walden: Or Life in the Woods.* Vintage, 1854.

Chapter V

Core moral values improve your sense of self

Self-definition continues throughout life ("I'm not the same person I was five years ago!"). It's part of personal growth. If you develop practices that help you define yourself—including but not limited to self-reflection—they will help you become thoughtful, aware, and the best version of yourself. This chapter focuses on developing core moral values, which you can apply when you want to be your best self, especially regarding how you affect other people. Adopting core moral values, a natural product of self-reflection, will improve your sense of self. *Living* such values allows you to experience yourself in ways that you admire and respect, and that enable you to positively assert yourself in the world.

Living morally should become a habit. You should just do it, without having to stop and think about it. Having good

values keeps you from having to reinvent a major part of yourself again and again, and from responding inappropriately
when—if your values had been in place—you'd have known
what to do right away.

We realize that the previous paragraphs use terms that may
seem elusive. What is a "sense of self"? What are "core moral
values"? You've probably heard these terms before, but we'd like
to define them in the context of young people's health and
wellness.

What is a sense of self?—Your sense of self is a measure of
who you think you are—a good, decent person, or a creep. If
you have core values that you respect, you will have a better
sense of self than if you know you are indifferent to other people and the planet (a sort of greed-is-good mentality that was
popular in the 1980s and '90s, but has since been debunked as
unworthy of anyone who should care about their place in the
community—which is everyone).

Psychologists often use the term "self-concept" for sense of
self. It's more expansive than what we've just outlined, and refers
to how a person perceives themselves *as a whole*, including their
unique identity, beliefs, strengths, weaknesses, and emotions,
as well as values. It's how we see ourselves in *context* with our
experiences and our current situation. From this perspective,
the definition could be stated simply as "our perception of the
characteristics that define us"—including everything from personal traits, likes and dislikes, belief system or moral code, on
down to whatever motivates us. Our self-concept is our unique
identity as a person. Having a "strong" self-concept means having a deep understanding of our identity and accepting it.

What are core moral values?—Core moral values are basic beliefs about how we want to live in the world and treat other people. They're "core" because they're fundamental, and central to our idea of who we are. Imagine yourself saying, for example,

- "I want to decelerate environmental damage by minimizing my use of plastics and forever chemicals."
- "I want to ensure that people less fortunate than I can get a fair shake."
- "I want to be kind to the people I date and never leave them feeling used and devalued."
- "I will pursue a profession that's not all about making money, where I can give back to society some measure of the benefits it's given me."

You probably can't imagine discarding this type of deeply held conviction—it just seems to reflect who you are. Your core values (like the ones above) help you be the person you want to be. If asked, you'd say, "I believe these things. They matter to me." This is how core moral values operate.

Developing a moral compass—How do we develop core moral values? In previous eras, people looked to religion, starting with the Ten Commandments (or whatever strictures their religion laid down). They prayed for guidance. Of course, they also relied on other sources—often family members or community leaders—and developed what was called a moral compass, a complex mix of values that seemed sanctioned by authority ("If Mother Teresa thinks this is the way to go, that's enough for me"). But more recently, as society has become less reliant on received wisdom, it's possible to find core values in an array of sources that seem compatible with who you'd like to be (independent of whether someone says you *ought* to be that way). Most people feel more comfortable relying on their own—necessarily informed—judgment, often spending time to reflect on values that they may adopt for the long term.

You may question the values available to you from some sources. In addition, values that seem right in most situations may seem inadequate in others. This is normal to value formation, which should not be unquestioning and should respond to life as you live it. Just don't rationalize your values in the interest of expediency ("I don't owe those people anything, so I don't have to consider their feelings"). Be honest with yourself and act accordingly. Still, your values may evolve. What seems right today may not seem so right a few years from now. You should feel comfortable in your values so that you can readily apply them. They should be in sync with the best version of yourself as only you can define it.

The point is to have core values that, when you reflect on them, make sense to you as workable in everyday situations. They can be aspirational, but not so aspirational that you get mad at yourself for always falling short. Like so much in life, choosing core values is a balancing act ("Can I *reasonably* be expected to apply these values?"). Some value systems—say, Marxism—are less forgiving than others. Your values, and your long-term adherence to them, will reflect the sources of those values.

Of course, you may have heard of doctrines such as situation ethics, which states that there are no moral rules or laws, and that the context of your action should determine how you act. Under this approach, the general guideline is that the correct action is the most loving action. There is much to be said for this approach. Still, it is not easily applied in an array of situations—for example, how you can best limit your carbon footprint in a crowded world. It merely tells you that you should limit it, which any genuinely ethical approach will tell you. While you might factor situation ethics into how (in some limited situations) you apply your core moral values, it's still crucial to have such values.

Finding good sources—Here are some sources of such values that you might turn to, which still include those that embody received wisdom (though not religion, since that is personal to you). In our current intellectual environment, where everything received is open to question, you have greater latitude than ever in making your choices. The sources discussed below are not exclusive; you can also decide which to consider most important. Finally, you'll recognize that *where* you acquire your values determines the *type* of values you acquire. For example, your family will impart different values—such as the need for sharing—than will a higher education based on the need for critical thinking.

Consider these for starters:

- *Your own experience*—For example, if someone you dated left you feeling hurt and devalued, you might decide—as a basic principle of your interpersonal relations—that you will never treat anyone else that way ("I know how I felt, and it was awful"). Your experience provides the basis for empathy with others. You can anticipate how they will feel. So, you decide to make it one of your core values that you'll never set them up to feel that way.

Your experience may also have exposed you to seeing how less fortunate people live. For example, over the summer break, you volunteered in a shelter for newly arrived migrants. It was jarring—the kids had no shoes, and families had to take turns sleeping in the few beds available. You decide that whatever career you choose, you will focus less on making money than on helping those less fortunate than you. Here, your impetus is not empathy—you don't lack basic necessities—but rather an appreciation for how, with your help, other people could lead better lives. You feel that you cannot ignore the need.

Your experience may expose you to problems that once seemed abstract until you see their effects in person. You know about environmental degradation, but once you see the mounds of plastic near a lake where your family vacations, you decide that you cannot allow this pollution to continue. You decide to do what you can to stop it, and this becomes a core moral value. You want to leave things better than how you found them.

- *Family*—Suppose you grew up with a brother and sister. You learned to share, and to support each other. You learned to cooperate. You learned that there is a type of intimacy, based on love, where nothing is

secret because you all want the same thing—to help
each other thrive and be happy. At home, you feel
safe. As you grow to maturity, "family togetherness"
emerges as a core value in your life ("I'm going to
build a nurturing family, just like the one I grew up
in"). Your family was an *example* of this value. You
perpetuate it, and set an example of it to your kids.

Suppose further that your parents imparted certain
values to you and your siblings, and they became
ingrained in you. Now you cannot imagine being
any other way. Your family was a source of *education*,
where values were not just exemplified but taught.

- *Formal education*—As you advance through school,
you are taught certain core values—"You live in your
body, so take care of it" may be one of them. It's a
value that this *Guide* seeks to reinforce. In college,
you may take courses that encourage you to think in
new ways—as a result, you develop new values ("I
never understood the Civil War before—it's inspired
me to care about equality"). Formal education is
designed to expand our awareness of the world and
to promote critical thinking. We learn not to just
take things for granted, and to investigate the sources
of information. Critical thinking itself may become
a core value ("I consider all sides before making up
my mind"). Likewise, we are exposed to the scientific
method—Prove everything!—and may decide that
we should apply it in a wider sphere (for example,
politics). Formal education can change us profoundly,

and allow us to form values that we could not have formed except through systematic exposure to new, challenging ideas.

- *Community*—You may become involved in your community by canvassing for a political party, volunteering at a nonprofit, or tutoring kids whose schools have fewer resources than yours. These activities encourage you to work for what is generally perceived as improving the quality of life of the people around you—or, in the case of politics, creating conditions that some segments of the populace think will make life better. In going out for these activities, you will likely absorb values. You will define yourself in reference to people you don't know well, but who matter to you as a collective with common interests. You may even become an activist, dedicated to bringing about social change through solidarity with members of the community who see the world as you do. Such solidarity, which can be emotionally satisfying, will reinforce the communally based values that you've developed.

- *Mentors*—Sometimes we work with or are related to people who are sources of good moral values. Sometimes we encounter a teacher or professor who, by example, enables us to see such values in action. These people can make a profound impression on us, since we experience at close range how their values are manifest—and can help change other people's lives for the better.

- *Leaders*—Some leaders, especially those of social movements, are a major source of values. We look up to them. Martin Luther King Jr., for example, was one of the great leaders of the twentieth century. His values still resonate ("Judge a man not by the color of his skin, but by the quality of his character"). Closer to our own time, Steve Jobs, the founder of Apple, arguably changed the world with the iPhone and the personal computer. Apple's motto, "Think different," is a fascinating example of how he shook things up. In its grammatical incorrectness, it conveys a core value: you can change anything for the better, provided you see it in a new light and free of preconceptions. Leaders inspire us to adopt their values.

- *Culture*—Our culture is the source of ideology, a complex of ideas that are not specifically enunciated because they are so pervasive that few people question them. Take capitalism, for example. In the US, we're all capitalists because we all want to buy and sell— we'll happily sell our work to the highest bidder so that we can purchase lots of stuff. Capitalism is the source of our values, even if we don't stop to think about it—work hard, pay for what you want, compete to earn as much as you can. We never stop to think that in other cultures, which are less capitalistic, these values may sound odd and even subversive.

  Yet even apart from ideology, culture is a source of all kinds of values—most of them glaringly visible. We absorb values from pop (popular) culture, such as

TikTok influencers and YouTube performers ("Thin is beautiful," "Start your own business to survive the next Depression"), and the singers who extol being faithful in love. On TV, in movies, and online, we see images that promote values ("Your clothes matter—they reflect your capacity to define the latest trends"). The quick availability of culturally based values (some good, some not so good) raises an important question: "How do I know which values to accept, and which to reject as inappropriate for me?" This is where self-reflection comes in.

The culture is also a source of received wisdom—for example, the idea that while democracy may be flawed, it's still the best way to govern a political entity and to give everyone a voice. Probably that's true. But in acquiring values, we learn to question aspects of those values even as we generally accept them. For example, we might say, "Democracy in general is great, but where there is no mechanism for equal voting rights, then we need to fix it." The takeaway is that it's tricky to absorb values from one's culture, which is a cacophony of voices and ideas. But culture is unavoidable, so we should exercise our best judgment when we engage with it.

Applying your values—Forming core moral values is a complicated process. There are so many potential sources that can exert an influence. To sort things out, it's fine to talk with people you trust. Just be sure that, in the end, the values you adopt are *your* values, not pronouncements that you repeat by rote for the sake of ease and social acceptance. Be sure that you have the will and ability to apply them. Of course, some values may be socially unacceptable (think of feminism a hundred years ago). But if you believe in them after careful and unbiased consideration, that's fine. You can base your sense of self on them.

When you choose core values, they're rarely generic ("I value kindness," "I value teamwork"). In most instances, they're your personalized *version* of such values ("I value kindness to animals," "I value teamwork at the office"). They reflect your own interests and concerns, even to the point where your version of kindness and teamwork may differ substantially from someone who also considers themselves kind (to elderly people) and a team player (who steals home so their baseball team can score). This is as it should be, since research shows that you're unlikely to follow through on abstract "values"—values have to matter to you, and be practicable. You should be able to live them.

Commonly recognized moral values—Some values are aspirational ("I hope to be a good team player") and can represent important goals. You can work toward them. But for purposes of strengthening your sense of self, it's important to be able to live your values—and live *with* your values—now. They should inform your choices. Here are some commonly recognized values that you can personalize and try to make your own. While you will certainly find others, these can jump-start your thinking:

- Integrity, accountability to others

- Authenticity ("what you see is what you get")
- Communication, a willingness to hold yourself available to others
- Dependability, so that other people can rely on you
- Empathy, a concern for others' feelings
- Excellence, always doing your best work
- Respect for others' autonomy
- Paying people who work for you a fair wage, based on their true worth
- Altruism and kindness, where your natural response is a concern for others
- Curiosity, not takings things for granted
- Critical thinking, so that you don't take information for granted
- Humility, where you recognize that (like everyone) you're imperfect
- Accepting responsibility for your mistakes
- Adaptability, a resistance to being rigid

These are just a few. You can take an inventory of your core values ("What *are* my values?" "Do I live them, or are they aspirational?" "Do I respect and admire them?" "Should I add more?"). Your values strengthen your sense of self by *defining* you as a moral actor in the world. Much of the time, our sense of self reflects how other people see us. If we know that they admire us, we're likely to admire ourselves. In this sense, moral values are like two-way mirrors, where we can watch people watching us. We act in accordance with how they seem to react toward us.

Some people may admire us for the wrong reasons ("That guy is a brilliant liar!"). This is why we need to use good judgment in choosing whose opinion should matter.

Following the two-way mirror analogy, consider how many of the bullet points above involve showing concern for *others*— not just "integrity, accountability to others," but also (to name just a few) "dependability," "respect for others' autonomy," and "paying people who work for you a fair wage." Concern for how you interact with and affect other people is crucial to developing sound core values. This does not in the least diminish your developing a sense of self. It just means that you'll function better among other people, without annoying or even angering them. Developing core moral values thus entails keeping others in your sights, which means keeping your *effect* on them in your sights.

But is any such concern simply altruistic (with no expected return), or even gratuitous (merely pointless)? No. People notice how we behave toward them. They care. If we adopt core moral values focused on creating good interactions—if not necessarily great relationships—we help create an environment where they are more likely to care about how they treat us.

How to use your sense of self—This chapter focuses on core moral values as the basis of a strong sense of self, rather than on all the factors (strengths, weaknesses, and emotions) that psychologists might use to describe your self-concept. This is because at your stage of development, good values are crucial— and it would take an entire book to examine all the other factors. However, in both our approach and the psychologists', *how you perceive yourself* is key. Do you respect your values and, by implication, yourself? Are you working toward defining the best moral values that you can, based on the demands of your life?

Because a sense of self is based on self-perception, having a strong sense of self (as opposed to one that's out of focus) means accepting yourself for who you are. That's not always easy when you know you're not your best self. It's rare that someone just says "I accept that I'm a lousy person" without trying to make improvements. Self-acceptance entails some measure of *approval* ("My values are sort of okay . . .") and doing what it takes to generate *continued* approval (". . . and I'm working on making them first-rate"). People with a strong sense of self, based on solid principles, are less likely to be bruised when they're criticized. For example, if someone says you didn't take enough responsibility for a mistake—implying that your values don't readily account for your role in society—you'll be more inclined to defend yourself effectively ("I did take responsibility, and besides, so did several other people"). Likewise, you may be more comfortable taking a risk because you know you'll be guided by good values.

On the other hand, people with a poor sense of self often have difficulty making decisions. They feel directionless and subject to intense self-criticism. They may lack self-esteem and the sense of purpose that good moral values provide. They feel as if they're not good enough. Cultivating your values, and the strong sense of self to which they contribute, can have important practical effects on how you perform and how other people see you.

Ultimately, you are building a repertoire of core moral values that will define you as you mature. As your circumstances change, you may refine these values, leave some behind, and emphasize some over others. That's fine. But sustaining a strong sense of self will depend, in no small part, on values you develop now and can start living (even though they may change). In this regard, our values can segue into habits, largely automatic responses that we don't have to reflect on as we're called to act in an array of situations. We just know what to do, and we do it. The value/habit connection is what makes us reliable moral actors. We're confident that we know what to do, so other people can be confident in us as well. Building strong, reliable moral values allows us to be the kind of person that others want to work with and, generally, be around.

Don't think of values as strictly personal ("They're my business, and not yours!"). They can also be viewed as social currency. They facilitate your relationships with people and allow these people to be confident in you. Forming good values is therefore a social as well as a personal necessity. It's part of participating in a civilized society—which, in this case, will also have a personal payoff.

Struggling with moral values—Sometimes we struggle. We aren't sure what we think or feel. We may think something is a moral issue—like sexual orientation, or gender identity—when it is profoundly determined by other factors beyond our control or understanding. In these cases, when there may be no right or wrong (but only what seems right or wrong for us), we should be honest with ourselves and with others. We should never struggle in silence. Find compatible people, or people you can trust, and talk through your issues. Find a supportive community. If you need professional help, get it.

Struggle is a form of personal growth. We emerge from the struggle as stronger individuals (note term "individuals"). In the struggle, we measure ourselves against received wisdom and other people's views and determine who we want to be.

If you have an array of core moral values and, as a result, a strong sense of self, your struggle with difficult issues will be *less* difficult. You'll be more likely to see yourself positively and not criticize yourself or feel helpless. Think of a strong sense of self as a defense against potentially debilitating impulses. We all need to feel strong, and a sense of self is a good place to start.

Takeaways—Core moral values are essential to a strong sense of self. They are basic to who we believe we are. We should therefore start developing our values now—we can turn to an array of sources to obtain them. But no matter where we locate our values, it's crucial that we make them our own. We should personalize our values so that we can live them. They should not be abstractions that we only nominally support. Core moral values will enable us to better navigate challenges as they arise.

Questions to ask yourself and to discuss:

- Am I working on developing core moral values, based on the array of sources available to me?
- Are my values sufficiently suited to me so that I can live them?
- Do I have a strong sense of myself, or am I mostly concerned just with fitting in, without giving too

much thought to how fitting in will affect the work I
am doing to define myself?

- Am I comfortable with myself as a moral actor in
  society, or do I need to improve?
- When I'm in a social setting, am I aware of how
  I affect other people—do they seem comfortable
  around me, or standoffish? If the latter, is it because I
  seem self-involved rather than interested in them and
  the world at large?
- Do I have to think hard before I take actions that
  affect others, or have I developed habitual responses
  that consider my effect on other people?

Further reading

Cole, William. *The ABC Formula: Building Your Life's Enduring
Core Values*. Authority Publishing, 2011.

Connors, Christopher. *The Value of You: The Guide to Living
Boldly and Joyfully Through the Power of Core Values*. Self
published, 2017.

Demartini, John. *The Values Factor: The Secret to Creating an
Inspired and Fulfilling Life*. Berkley, 2013.

Rifenbary, Jay. *No Excuse! Incorporating Core Values,
Accountability, and Balance into Your Life and Career*.
Possibility Press, 2014.

Schelske, Mark Alan. *Discovering Your Authentic Core Values: A
Step-by-Step Guide*. Live210 Media, 2012.

Chapter VI

Healthy relationships are integral to your well-being

We live in an interconnected world, where almost everything we do involves other people. In this sense, we are always creating potential relationships—some casual and fleeting, others verging on the profound. As John Donne observed four centuries ago, "No man is an island." We all engage with each other. In some cases, we just act *toward* these others (with whom we are passively partnered), while in others there can be intense, continuous interaction. Thus, at any point in space and time, this island-less world is crisscrossed with billions of lines, each representing a human exchange. This chapter will discuss how—and whether—we should integrate these relationships into our lives. What sorts of relationships work for us, and how do we cultivate them?

The skills we acquire in developing and maintaining relationships are crucial. We will naturally refine them as we mature, but it's important to start acquiring them now. **What are healthy relationships?**—We tend to think of a relationship as intimate and romantic, but there are all kinds of relationships, and we should have an array of them. Good friends can help us sort out our problems. They can be there to help us have fun. Even casual friends are important, since you never know what you'll learn from someone. We should practice making connections because the world runs on who you know (if you're well connected, it's easier to find a job). More importantly, some friends that we make as young people will stay with us forever. They will grow with us, and share our ups and downs. Their advice—and company—can be invaluable just because they understand us. We won't have to start from scratch and explain ourselves when all we want is the comfort of someone who knows what to say.

Let's consider some of the various kinds of relationships that we develop. The first relationships that anyone forms are within the family.

Family relationships—Unlike other relationships discussed in this chapter, family relationships are not discretionary. We *choose* our friends and romantic partners, but we're born into our families. We're related to them forever. At least as teenagers, we live with those people. Our parents support us. We can't just say, "Too bad, I'm outta here." The expectations are different.

Family relationships can be difficult. They can make you feel disempowered. They can make you feel like no one's listening. But there's also the flip side.

Families have the *potential* to teach us how to relate to others. They can serve as templates for demonstrating generosity, compromise, empathy, in fact most of the personal qualities that we'll need to form relationships outside the family. If your family is even moderately functional—that is, if everyone loves each other, even if they don't quite understand you—you can acquire skills that will help you relate to your friends and romantic partners.

From our parents and siblings, it's possible to learn unconditional love. We learn how to give advice and criticize without antagonism. We learn to give and receive without keeping score. In this sense, family helps us grow beyond the limitations of our ego. It initiates us into the world of other people, with whom we *must* get along if we're going to succeed.

Ultimately, we may value our own intimate relationships more than our birth family. Our friendships may become our new, intentional family. That's okay. But right now, while you're still in your birth family, try to make the most of it. Practice empathy. Practice compromise. Much of it will just come naturally. You should pay attention to those inclinations, since you'll want to call on them in all your relationships.

Intimate relationships—Everyone wants to be in love. It's fun and exciting. Our society glorifies it. But if we embark on an intimate, romantic relationship, what should we expect? That is not the same question as "What should we settle for?" which diminishes the person who is settling (as well as the person we're settling for). The first rule of romantic partnering is that both parties should feel equal. Both should feel loved, respected, and able to trust the other. When there are issues, neither should be afraid to raise them, and both should be able to expect an honest, conscientious response. Neither should be so locked into their own concerns that they're unwilling to forgive and work things out.

But the impulse to love can feel irresistible. Sometimes we just *want* to be in love, and the idea is so attractive (even apart from the person we choose to be in love with) that we don't stop to consider all the ramifications of committing ourselves to an intense, mind-bending experience with *that person*. We want to give in to the hormonal rush and ride the wave of ecstasy.

The hormonal effects of love are real. Falling in love can trigger the release of dopamine, also known as the "feel-good" hormone, which is associated with pleasure, enthusiasm, and motivation. High levels of dopamine can make us feel giddy, energetic, and euphoric, even to the point where we lose our appetite and ability to sleep. Love can also trigger the release of oxytocin, which causes feelings of contentment, calmness, and security. Our hormones act to reinforce the desire to stay bonded to the object of our love, an evolutionary mechanism to ensure that offspring resulting from that bond have a supportive family structure. If there ever was a mind/body nexus, love is Exhibit A.

But think for a moment. Are we just passive participants in a grand evolutionary scheme, destined to fall in love even if we wind up in some modern version of *Romeo and Juliet*? Of course not. Recall Daniel Kahneman's *Thinking, Fast and Slow*, discussed in Chapter I. Kahneman would say, "When you're about to enter a romantic relationship, slow down and think about it." Ask questions (not just of yourself, but of your friends). Consider the relationship's pros and cons. Are you really that compatible, apart from the initial sexual attraction which—admittedly—can just blow you away?

You probably don't want to ask such questions. You probably think they could sully something wonderful. To the extent that you do ask them, you probably respond with, "I don't want to mess things up by seeming scared or overly cautious. I don't want to seem like I don't truly love this person and accept them despite their potential faults. I don't want to seem reluctant to give myself to the relationship." But in some other part of your brain, you probably know that those responses are wrong. If nothing else, allow your instinct for self-preservation to kick in. Find some happy medium between fight or flight. Slow down, at least initially.

Timing is everything when you start a relationship. Maybe you go on a couple of dates, and then there it is: SEX. "I don't really know this person, but I like them, so why not?" You may even feel that sex will move the relationship in the right direction. The problem is that once you have sex, the nature of the relationship changes. There are expectations, not just for more sex, but for a degree of closeness that—for whatever reason—may make you uncomfortable. There may be expectations of exclusivity when, in fact, you want to date other people. *Unmet expectations can lead to hurt.* They can cause misunderstandings and arguments, which can lead to still more hurt. None of this is good for your head.

So, what's the answer? Romantic relationships without sex may not seem very romantic. But especially in the case of teenagers, romance depends on both partners' comfort levels because one partner may not yet be ready for sex. If they're not, then the other shouldn't exert pressure (and by the way, in hetero-, same-sex, and nonbinary relationships, pressure can be exerted in both directions). Sex also comes in many forms, and—at different stages of a relationship—some may feel more appropriate than others. It's okay to stop with some forms, leaving others for another time. When you consider that young men in the United States start having intercourse at an average of 16.8 years of age, and young women at 17.2 years, there seems to be an awful lot of time before you go all the way.

You might feel that negotiating over what is and isn't appropriate makes sex feel less sexy. You may not want to turn sex into what feels like a transaction. But remember, sex is powerful. Orgasms release oxytocin, which not only makes you feel happy but also promotes the desire to bond with the other person. *Sex makes you want more sex with the person with whom you had sex.* The answer to "What am I supposed to do about sex?" is complicated. But here are four up-front rules to consider before we examine how to form relationships that will lead to a sexual involvement where both partners are comfortable.

- Never exert pressure on anyone to have sex—it can lead to hurt and recriminations, and even destroy a relationship that may have been promising. (It's not okay to say, "Let's just get sex out of the way, so we can think about the rest of our relationship"—that is exactly the reverse of how things should go.)

- You have the right to consent (or not to consent) to a request for sex, and your unwillingness to provide it should be definitive. If the other person tries to pressure you, they have crossed a red line and shown their lack of respect for you. Probably you should end the relationship.

- No matter how difficult it may seem, you owe it to yourself not to rush into sex, even if it's consensual. It's even more difficult to turn back once you've had sex, short of just ending the relationship entirely.

- If someone cares about you—as *you*, and not just as a sex object—they'll wait for sex to develop at a pace that feels natural (to you), rather than treating it as some biological necessity or as something that "everybody" does.

What should we expect from a relationship? Notice that we didn't say "romantic" relationship because not all relationships end up in romance—that is, in what we experience as love. Nor should the possibility of sex be the goal of becoming more than casual friends ("I'm dating this person to find out if I'm interested enough to have sex"). We should expect good communication, respect, trust, fairness, and honesty—among other qualities. Most of these should be present from the start. Trust develops over time.

You might say, "I can't be bothered with any of this. I'm just interested in sex for its own sake." That's the hook-up mentality. But surprise, surprise. One partner often finds themselves wanting more, even while the other resists. It's a recipe for humiliation. You probably shouldn't try it, even if many of your friends are in relationships and you think, "Well, I should do *something*!" It's better to wait until you feel good about the person you're dating.

Also, it's important to ask yourself whether you feel ready for a romantic relationship. Maybe you just feel like dating several people, without making a commitment. It's fine. When you're ready, you're ready, and you don't have to justify yourself to anyone.

It's also important to realize that romantic relationships are not just about having fun. Teenagers' emotions can be turbulent, and their partners should recognize (and, ideally, accommodate) that. The point is to be there for each other. If sex happens, engage in it carefully, not just in terms of its emotional impact, but also by:

- Using protection to avoid an STD
- Making sure to use reliable birth control

Remember, there is no such thing as "it can't happen the first time." It can. Get advice from a nurse or a doctor before you do anything. You can learn a lot about life through a relationship—just be sure you approach it with care and a healthy concern for your own well-being.

Important qualities in any relationship—Suppose you *are* interested in starting a relationship, or maybe just starting a friendship that may or may not lead to romance. Or suppose you just want to make the most of your family relationships. Here are some qualities to look for.

- *Communication*—The process of sharing thoughts, feelings, and needs with a partner. It's a vital part of keeping a connection strong and can help preventing disagreements from escalating into argument. Poor communication can lead to feelings of isolation, anger, and sadness.

- *Respect*—Treating each other with dignity and valuing each other's opinions and feelings. It's the opposite of controlling someone and making them do what you want them to do.

- *Honesty*—Being authentic and transparent with your partner, in big and small ways. They shouldn't hide stuff!

- *Trust*—A feeling of security and confidence that allows people to be vulnerable and open to each other without fear of hurt or violation. Key elements include honesty, empathy, reliability, and support.

- *Fairness*—Treating your partner as an equal and working toward the needs of the relationship. It's about recognizing and respecting each person's needs (even though sometimes one person's needs may be more acute than the others'—eventually the pendulum will swing back).

- *Comfort*—Being able to be yourself around someone, to have different opinions, and to not feel pressured to do what you don't want to. You don't feel self-conscious. Emotional support is a key element.

- *Sharing*—A willingness to face problems together, and to participate in common experiences. It's not "I have my life and you have yours—so, good luck with what you're doing." Sharing often leads to compromise, the willingness of each party to meet somewhere in the middle when deciding what to do.

- *Generosity of spirit*—This is an inclination to share freely, joyously, and willingly. It's doing more than expected, acting with kindness, and sharing without any expectation of receiving something in return.
- *No narcissists!*—You don't want someone so concerned with themselves that they always put their needs ahead of yours and treat you as an afterthought. These people are toxic to your sense of self and will make you feel devalued.

In general, when you're contemplating any kind of relationship, look for someone with emotional intelligence—the ability to both manage their own emotions and understand yours. They should be responsive to you, not locked inside themselves or just too lazy to care. You'll probably be able to gauge someone's emotional intelligence fairly quickly (though beware of people who are initially on their best behavior, only to fall away from that standard sometime later).

Friendships—Friendships come in all sorts of flavors: from casual and transitory to intense and long-standing. It's as important to have friends, throughout our lives, as it is to be in love. When we're not in love, it can feel more important ("Oh, I have to tell you why we broke up, or I'll scream!"). But what makes a friend? If you look at the list of qualities that make someone a good romantic partner, then you'll have some answers. You can trust friends. They're reliable. They give you advice that's not self-interested. They're there when you need them.

Even if someone isn't a close friend, they're somewhere on our wavelength and that's what matters. They're *interested* in us, at least to a degree. A portion of their energy flows in our direction—not all the time, but enough so that we wouldn't choose to be without it. These may be people on the periphery of lives (we chat with them on the bus, or at the coffee shop after school). But slowly we build up a repertoire of topics ("Hey, check out that new vintage store!" "Did you hear that AI will be introduced in our coding class? "). There's a palpable mutuality which, though fleeting, returns again and again and sometimes even deepens. We couldn't do without these bursts of friendship to reassure us that we can connect in all sorts of ways.

At the opposite end of the spectrum are our long-standing friends. As with those on the periphery of our lives, there may still be only intermittent contact, but it's gone on for such a long time that we don't have to explain ourselves. When, for example, we bring up an issue with a sibling, we don't have to describe how it started. Our friends already know. We can dive right into the current situation. Nor do we need to justify ourselves, because our friends have already assured us of their sympathy to how we see things. Long-standing friends are a real comfort when we feel stressed. We should cultivate them.

Have we finally cleared the subject of sexuality? Sex is not a factor in most friendships. Okay, there are so-called "friends with benefits," where the sex is casual and no one expects much more. If both partners agree on the terms, these types of friends can still be supportive. You can still have fun with them. The risk is that this equilibrium may not be stable. Someone may decide that they want something more. They may become jealous. If you do enter this kind of friendship, be sure that's what you want. Be sure you can handle it if someone changes their mind.

But in every case, it's important to maintain a friendship. Friends can drift apart. We can't take friends for granted, assuming they'll be there when we need them. Keep in touch with your friends. Be curious ("What have you been up to lately?"). Share experiences ("Hey, my family's going hiking this weekend—would you like to join?"). Just let them know that you're thinking about them. When you have news ("I was finally able to get those braces off my teeth!"), share it. But be careful of your friends' feelings. If you know they might feel bad because you got into an Ivy and they didn't, let them know casually— don't call them and announce, "I'm deciding between Yale and Princeton—I don't know what to do!"

It's important to make enough time for friends. No one wants to feel that you're "fitting them in" between soccer practice and flute lessons. If there are things you both like to do— perhaps in-line skating or picking apples at upstate farms— then arrange an outing, with time to catch up afterward. Sure, everybody's busy, but when you think of all the interstitial time you spend on social media or watching sports, you can probably find more time than you think.

One way to cultivate friends is to be a good listener. Sometimes people just need to talk. It may be more important than any advice that you can give them. They may not even want your advice. They just want to feel they're not alone, and that someone understands them. You just need to show sympathy ("I realize how hard it is to lose your grandmother—my heart goes out to you"). Also, don't be afraid to show your own vulnerability. If people feel that you're sharing yourself with them, they'll want to reciprocate.

Another way to cultivate friends is to provide information they can use. For example, if you've heard of a great source of summer jobs, and you know your friend is looking, then tell them about it. As we mature, information is in many ways the currency of friendship, as people form networks and help each other get a leg up.

It's also important to laugh together. Don't just relate canned jokes, which anyone can do, but find things that are unique and share them ("Did you see those wild new dresses in Saks's windows? How could anyone *wear* them?"). Your friend will appreciate that you understood how funny they'd find such an observation. It suggests that you understand them. The point is to make your friends realize that they're part of your world. You don't take them for granted or treat them transactionally.

In this regard, never keep score with your friends. Sometimes you may do stuff for them, while other times they may do stuff for you. It's not always in equal proportion. It doesn't have to be. If people care about each other, that's what counts. We need to feel that despite all the chaos in the world, there is still a sphere where we can feel safe, understood, and even cherished. Friends populate this sphere, and they can stay with us for a long time, even as our respective lives change (often dramatically). That's huge, and crucial to our well-being.

Of course, even though we value our friends and treat them all with respect and kindness, we have different friends for different reasons. Some may be great cooks and would love to help us prepare a dinner for our parents' anniversary. Others may be skiers and would gladly accompany us on the slopes. Still others may want to solve the Sunday crossword with us. They understand the nature of the friendship so that, for example, the skier won't be offended if we don't invite them to help us cook. Nor should we be offended when the situation is reversed. Friends give each other what they can, and that's fine. The point is to maintain the friendship so that each one still feels like giving.

Sometimes we feel that what we give is unique, and we want our friends to respond in kind. For example, we may expose our vulnerable side ("I'm so scared of getting involved with someone who's so popular") and want to start a conversation about navigating our issues. While that's fine, and even a means of getting closer to someone, we should be careful not to make the other person feel overwhelmed by our issues. We should be careful not to make them feel that we expect them to disclose their own vulnerabilities. Every friendship has its rhythm. Don't rush or push things. Though we want our friends to feel generous toward us, we don't want them to feel that we expect more than they can give. Allow your friendships to grow at a pace that seems comfortable to everyone. Pay attention to how people react. If there is enough commonality and goodwill, the friendship will grow at the pace that it should.

Choosing the right people—don't hang out with the wrong ones—Not all potential friendships or relationships are good for us. Some people are just incompatible with our needs, our personalities, and our highest sense of ourselves. In some cases, their influence can be harmful ("Hey, I know where we can get some uppers"). A narcissistic person can make us feel small and unimportant. We should develop the skills—and the courage—to put distance between these people and ourselves. Just because they may be popular does not make them right for us. Though we may experience FOMO if we walk away, we'll be helping ourselves in the long run.

Earlier in this chapter, we listed several traits that define a good romantic partner and, by extension, a good friend. You'll probably encounter the opposite of these traits (dishonesty, lack of fairness, narcissism) in people whom you shouldn't hang out with. Such traits may not all be present, and you can always forgive a few lapses. But if you sense that people consistently behave in ways that set you edge, then you should probably not become (or remain) involved with them.

Apart from these obvious concerns, here are a few more flashing yellow lights when it comes to choosing people who are not right for you.

- They make fun of or belittle your commitments ("I like volunteering at the shelter for new immigrants, but they keep saying it's beneath me").
- They are jealous or resentful of your other friends and want to monopolize all your time and attention ("Hey, you and I are better than those clods, so let's

form our own little duo")—often, they feel inferior and need your affirmation to raise their self-esteem.
- They're manipulative and often find devious ways to make you be what they want and do what they want.
- They're competitive and try to one-up you in conversation or generally seem better than you—it may sometimes feel like they're just joking ("Hey, don't listen to my dumb friend"), but if it happens enough, you'll know they're not.
- They're hypercritical and always insisting that whatever you do is never good enough—probably they need to prove to themselves that they're better than you.
- They insist on doing everything their way and never want to compromise—sometimes they don't want to do anything that you want to do, and if they don't get their way, they'll take all their marbles and go home.

You can probably think of more traits that leave you feeling worn out, diminished, misunderstood, and unappreciated. If you start feeling that way around some people, then give them a wide berth. Just say something like "We're not making each other comfortable, so let's just try other people." If they keep coming around, you can repeat the same message until they get the point.

Of course, some people don't just get on your nerves and ruin your day. They are totally toxic, and you should conscientiously avoid them. These might include people who . . .

- *discourage you from doing your best work at school.* They might say, "Hey, let's cut classes today and take the train to New York." They might even add, "I know some twenty-four-hour parties with college kids that we can crash."

- *have friends make you nervous.* They may introduce you to people you'd never choose on your own, and who do things you don't want to do.

- *do drugs, drink to excess, and suggest that you join them.* These people are *dangerous*, and possibly even criminal.

- *ask you for money.* It's okay to borrow a few dollars occasionally, but not to ask for considerable sums— even when there's a promise to pay it back "soon." You don't know what the money will be used for, even if they tell you where it's supposedly going. You could wind up being implicated in some criminal activity or—at best—just losing your funds.

- *engage in sexting, and other risky social media activity.* You never want to meet up with people who practice sexting (sending sexually suggestive or even explicit messages through social media). They are likely disturbed.

Again, this list is far from complete. But it should encourage you to think about the compatibility of the people you meet, including those who make a point of meeting you. There are plenty of great people in the world, so just avoid those who can harm you. Just say something like, "I'm really not interested in taking our acquaintance any further, so I am going to stop it right here." If they persist, tell them again. You need to protect yourself.

Combat loneliness—In 2023, the surgeon general of the United States diagnosed an "epidemic" of loneliness (his advisory is cited in the Further Reading section at the end of this chapter). We're lonely because we're so mobile; families are smaller and more dispersed; it's harder to make new friends as we age (we're set in our ways and less likely to reach out to those who have grown in different directions). The advisory stated: "Loneliness and isolation represent profound threats to our health and well-being."

It went on to discuss the depression that results from loneliness, as well as the increased risk of heart disease, stroke, and dementia later in life. To prevent these effects, it proposed a national strategy to advance social connection, with projects from strengthening our social infrastructure with parks, libraries, and other places where people can meet, to reforming the digital environment so that our interactions with technology do not detract from meaningful connections with others.

Of course, we all feel lonely sometimes. But persistent, aching loneliness can leave us feeling as if no one knows or cares about us. We wonder how much we're really worth. So, as the Surgeon General recognizes, we should take positive action *on behalf of ourselves and each other* to keep loneliness from damaging our well-being.

This chapter has examined the importance of making friends. Even casual friends can make a big difference—we might not invite them to dinner, but they're great to meet for a walk in the park. They're great to catch up with periodically. They make us feel like we're in the world, rather than withdrawn into ourselves.

Cultivate friendships now. Try to avoid forming cliques and closed little groups. In the short run, they may make you feel superior, but they will ultimately isolate you from other people. They will discourage other people from approaching you. Most of the experiences we have in life are through other people, so make strong connections now. The idea is to share one's life and thoughts with other people. Involve them in our adventures, big and small. Friends can last a lifetime, and they make our lives much happier along the way.

You can also engage in activities where you can meet people you might like. If you are interested in ballroom dancing, take some lessons. If you like chess, join a local chess club. Maybe you'd like to go to the monthly meet-and-greet with authors at the local bookstore. You can even join an amateur theater production. The point is to put yourself in the way of people—congenial, compatible people who may be looking for someone just like you. You'll be on nonthreatening turf where, at the very least, you can relax and have fun. You never know when you'll get lucky!

Solitude—While this chapter has focused on forming and maintaining relationships, we should also cultivate solitude—the state of being productively alone—which is different from feeling lonely. Solitude is the basis of mindfulness (Chapter III) and self-reflection (Chapter IV). It gives us a chance to catch up with ourselves outside the whirl of everyone else. Maybe we can read, bake bread, explore the city spontaneously. We can listen to music on our own personal playlist. We don't have to apologize to anyone for anything.

Since we're usually so busy, solitude is actually a luxury. But it's important to find time for it, since it helps us develop into who we want to be. Maybe it's practicing on the unicycle, or skateboarding, or juggling—or anything—outside everyone's gaze. Solitude is a source of freedom. We don't have to be self-conscious. It's a time when we can make things up as we go along; we can allow ourselves to fail and try to perfect things. We might even have fun.

We should never be afraid to be alone. On a good day, we can even turn loneliness into solitude by finding something productive to do. While solitude can never replace loneliness on a regular basis, it can make us feel more purposeful and engaged ("I'm baking ciabatta for the first time, and I'll give it to people if it turns out well"). The point is to cultivate a capacity for solitude and make the most of it.

Takeaways—Before getting involved romantically, think about whether the relationship feels right. Ask yourself questions. Don't rush into anything until you're sure. On the other hand, friendships are always crucial to our well-being. We should cultivate an array of different kinds of friends and try as hard as we can not to fall into loneliness. Friends can last forever, and our oldest ones can be real treasures. Nonetheless, we should make sure that we never get involved with people who may seem like friends but can harm us. We need to protect ourselves.

Questions to ask yourself and to discuss:

- Do I really want a romantic relationship, and am I ready to enter one?

- Have I sufficiently thought about the person I may become involved with romantically?
- Do I have different sorts of friends, so that someone will always be available no matter how I'd like to spend my time?
- Am I taking steps to both meet new people and keep up with the friends that I have?
- Do I treat my friends with kindness and respect and make enough time for them?
- Are there people in my social circle whom I should avoid?
- Am I comfortable with solitude?

Further reading

Aguirre, Leah, and Geraldine O'Sullivan. *The Girl's Guide to Relationships, Sexuality, and Consent: Tools to Help Teens Stay Safe, Empowered, and Confident.* Instant Help, 2022.

Friedberg, Ahron, MD, with Sandra Sherman. *Towards Happiness: A Psychoanalytic Approach to Finding Your Way.* Routledge, 2022.

Lang, Jennifer, MD. *Consent: The New Rules of Sex Education— Every Teen's Guide to Healthy Sexual Relationships.* Callisto Teens, 2018.

Murthy, Vivek, MD. "Our Epidemic of Loneliness and Isolation." US Surgeon General, 2023. https://www.hhs .gov/sites/default/files/surgeon-general-social-connection -advisory.pdf.

Riley, Rhodes. *Sex Education for Teenagers: Answers to Questions You Don't Want to Ask Your Parents About Puberty, Dating, and Staying Safe.* Self published, 2023.

Ornstein, Peggy. *Boys & Sex: Young Men on Hookups, Love, Porn, Consent, and Navigating the New Masculinity.* Harper, 2021.

Chapter VII

Empathy is essential to caring about each other

We often teach people to be what they already are. For example, while we tell everyone to show kindness, neuroscience shows that we are naturally inclined to help others—even when we don't know them. In *The Altruistic Brain: How We are Naturally Good*, Donald Pfaff describes brain mechanisms that propel us toward making life better for others, whether they need simple favors (like the woman negotiating subway stairs with a baby carriage) or a gargantuan gesture that could save their lives (like donating a kidney). The same is true of urging people to show empathy, which is basically a type of shared understanding ("I know how you feel about losing your pet—I had the same experience, and I'm here for you"). We're inclined that way already.

Yet even though science knows that we are inclined toward empathy, this is one of those all-things-being-equal ideas with a million real-life exceptions ("Maybe I empathize with that person, but I'm too busy to go out of my way to show it"). We find excuses. We subordinate our natural inclinations to mundane considerations. This is why advocating for empathy, though paradoxical at some theoretical level, still makes sense. It's important to demonstrate why empathy is important. It makes the world a more civilized place. It makes *you* more civilized, and able to get on in an environment where people judge you by how you behave ("Oh, he's so self-involved—he never lifts a finger for anyone"). It even makes you like yourself better ("I'm glad I showed my support when my neighbor lost her husband—I know it made a difference to her").

This chapter concerns why you should push past any immediate resistance and tap into your natural impulse to empathize. It's about why empathy is valuable. Society developed because humans naturally cooperate and respond to each other's needs. The Tower of Babel story is about what happens when people fail to cooperate—things fall apart. We should think about how showing empathy can become a habit, which we practice without weighing all the competing options ("I'll leave empathy to that woman's family/colleagues/bridge club") except when our own needs literally prevent us. We should think about how, as a habit, empathy is an important element of our future selves—especially as we work to become the best version of ourselves.

What is empathy?—Thinking of empathy as an *awareness* of other people's emotions is a good place to start. In most areas of life, we naturally *want* to be aware. We want to align our senses with the reality around us (which is why crossing the street with your head in your phone is unnatural). This desire for perceptual clarity should be no different when it comes to people's feelings. The impulse to protect ourselves from reality ("I don't want to see, or hear, or think about how they feel—it's too upsetting") is short-sighted. Just as we process our own feelings by means of self-reflection, we should engage with others' feelings. Of course, someone may say, "You'll never understand what I feel, so I don't want your empathy". But if you're tactful ("To the extent that I can understand, I empathize"), you'll be received as caring, as opposed to self-absorbed. You will have made a connection.

One further note. You might ask, "What is the difference between empathy and sympathy?" Empathy is the ability to understand how someone feels, while sympathy displays our relief at not having similar problems. Some people can sympathize but not empathize. It's generally better, from a social perspective, to show empathy. Empathy creates an immediate connection. The language is different ("I understand how you feel" vs. "I'm sorry for your loss"). People can sense the difference. You can sense the difference. So, try to empathize. Later, this chapter will discuss how to become more empathetic.

How can I practice empathy?—Empathy means that you feel what someone else feels. You understand what they are experiencing in terms that relate to you: "Oh, you just lost your mother—I'd be distraught if that happened to me." You don't actually need to have suffered through the same events that they have, but you need to be able to relate to their feelings. Either through imagination or by recalling an analogous experience, you calibrate your feelings to theirs. In this case, though your mother is still alive, you recall how you felt when your grandmother died. If you can't find a close analogy in your own experience, then you can think through the stories you've heard of loss and imagine yourself a protagonist in them. Sooner or later, you'll be able to put yourself in the place of the person with whom you should empathize. Just listening to them describe their feelings may trigger an empathetic response.

But empathy is not just about resonating with someone's grief. You can empathize with their positive experiences ("Oh, you met someone—I remember how great I felt when I met someone!"). In this sense, empathy is an agile, expansive feeling. It allows you to reach out and connect with people in an array of contexts. You just need to identify the occasions—if they don't jump right out at you. Empathy comes down to awareness, being alive to the world rather than submerged in yourself.

In social settings, if you *feel* empathy, then express it. Empathy that is bottled up will not make a difference. It should be externalized so that the object of your empathy benefits, ideally by knowing how you feel. In this sense, empathy is instrumental. It affects human relations. By extension, even when there's no way to tell people how you feel—for example, when they're fleeing a war zone—that's still no reason to stifle your emotion. Just holding these victims in your mind ("I couldn't survive if I were homeless") will make you feel better. You *know* that you care; you're not the sort of person who'd dismiss the events as none of your business. You may even be empowered to act remotely, perhaps by supporting relief agencies. That would be another way of showing empathy and making it an instrument of outreach to others. *You'll* feel good, even if other people can't personally thank you.

Psychologists have shown that by helping us *feel* connected to others, empathy promotes a sense of well-being. People who empathize more often report greater happiness, especially when they empathize with others' positive feelings. Ever wonder why charities like the Red Cross show people smiling in a disaster? It's to make you feel "I'm so happy they found some relief—I'll help them keep smiling!" Charity gets us to empathize and externalize the feeling. Consider the three kinds of empathy which, though distinct, often occur in stages as part of the *process* of empathizing.

- *Cognitive empathy*—This is our ability to identify and understand other people's emotions. It is primarily a thought process and is not the same as feeling what they feel.
- *Emotional empathy*—This is when you emotionally, and perhaps even physically, feel what another person is experiencing. As emotional contagion, it helps us respond to others' pain on a visceral level (Bill Clinton famously remarked, "I feel your pain." That was a literal expression of emotional empathy). In the caring professions (and perhaps Clinton saw the presidency as one of them), it is essential.
- *Compassionate empathy*—This allows us not only to understand and feel what another person is experiencing, but to help that person. It's when empathy is externalized.

To fully experience empathy, we move through each stage—first understanding, then feeling, then doing something about what we understand and feel. For example, suppose your friend just experienced a breakup with someone, and is worried that they'll never meet anyone as wonderful again. They blame themselves ("I blew it. I should have been more attentive when they needed my support"). So, first you try to understand their problem—a sense of loss, a sense that they made a mess of things. Then you try to feel what they do—real pain, as well as disappointment in themselves. Finally, you do something to help—you might say, "I get it, but you shouldn't blame yourself. You're a kind and decent person. At the time, you did what seemed right, even though they decided that they needed more." This shows your friend that you understand what happened, you put yourself in their shoes, and that you thought through the events with compassion. You're on their side emotionally.

The exchange can bring you and your friend closer. You've literally shared an important experience—you weren't just present after the fact as an objective analyst; you also relived the experience on a subjective level, so that your advice and support reflected your emotional grasp of the situation and willingness to help. As a result of your close-in engagement, your friend may feel buoyed. They may start feeling better about themselves and, finally, start looking for another relationship sooner and with greater confidence. *You* get to feel valuable, as if you've made a difference in someone's life when they needed you.

Empathy is a two-way street. While you don't expect someone to compensate you ("You helped me, so I'm buying you dinner"), you still derive great personal satisfaction from having helped. Maybe your self-esteem increases. Maybe your relationship with the person you helped becomes stronger. In this sense, empathy is a two-way street with no defined end. Rather, it's about how you feel about yourself going forward, and how other people feel about you. Imagine the alternative if you hadn't shown your friend empathy. You would have seen them continue to suffer and blame themselves, and you would not have benefited personally from your response. From this perspective, your display of empathy was a pretty good investment in your own well-being. It strengthened your social connection.

Empathy is important for well-being—Perhaps, as your friend reflects on how deftly you displayed empathy, they may think, "I wish I had been as empathetic, and possibly saved my relationship." Maybe they hadn't cleared all the obstacles to showing empathy. Maybe they didn't understand the gravity of the other person's need (a failure of cognitive empathy). Empathy takes practice—we may be able to empathize with people whose need is obvious ("Oh, you lost your grandmother"), but not so able when the need is subtler, as it may have been in the context of your friend's partner. It's important to consider the benefits of empathy so that we don't act casually about it.

- *Relationships depend on empathy*—As in the anecdote above, empathy is crucial to romantic as well as platonic relationships. It draws people together through shared understanding and helps keep us from feeling alone.
- *Empathy helps situate us in the world*—If we respond to events around us with empathy, we feel like we

are engaged (even if we can't directly do much about those events). We feel like we're not just hiding in a cocoon, which, eventually, can lead to feelings of guilt.

- *We're less depressed and anxious when we display empathy*—While empathy may impose costs in terms of our time and emotional capital ("How am I supposed to care about someone when I've got so much going on?"), research demonstrates that it helps alleviate anxiety and reduce depression. Perhaps this is because we feel less alone, less like the only person with problems.

- *Empathy is necessary to team building and leadership*— If we want people to work with us, they should feel that we understand their interests and care about their needs. No one will commit to a project if they feel like a cog in our machine—they need to feel connected with us in real-life terms. If we are in business, clients expect us to anticipate and respond to their concerns.

- *If you are skilled at displaying empathy, you become known as the go-to person in your group*—Word gets around. If you become known as someone who takes time for others, people will seek out your friendship. In this sense, empathy has a knock-on effect. It keeps paying you back in terms of the regard that others show you.

- *Writers need empathy*—If you write fiction, you need to get inside your characters' heads and figure out why they should act one way or another. But no matter what you write, you should anticipate your readers' expectations and likely reactions. By imagining a likely reader, you can (figuratively) interrogate them: what will they be drawn to, what will make them turn the page?

- *The earth needs empathy*—Increasingly, philosophers as well as activists have begun to argue that the same empathy that defines our human-to-human relationships should define our relationship to the earth. The idea is that if we appreciate the earth's fragility, and understand how fragile we ourselves can be, then we'll respond to climate change and the environment's continued decline.

The question becomes, how do we become more empathetic? How do we cultivate empathy as a skill, and then make it a habit?

Cultivating empathy—This chapter began by observing that empathy is innate to human beings, but sometimes you'd never know it. Either a million reasons arise for not showing empathy ("I'm so busy," "I don't understand the situation," "If I extend myself, they'll only want more"), or we just aren't sure how to *be* empathetic. Here are some suggestions.

- *When you find yourself making excuses, try to get past them*—Consider, for example, your fear of becoming emotionally involved. This is a legitimate concern, for example, if you know someone as an acquaintance but want to keep things at that level.

You don't want to be drawn into their lives or risk their becoming emotionally dependent. As a result, you just play it safe—you do nothing, even though you feel bad on their account. But wait! You could still respond, but keep things simple, perhaps by sending a note or a text (though don't make pro forma offers of help that you know will be refused). If they're a chocoholic, you could send a fancy box of bonbons. The point is to let them know you care, even if it's in proportion to the type of relationship that you have with them.

If you have other reasons for not acting ("I'm just too busy"), try to imagine how you would feel if someone said that when you were hurting. You'll probably end up finding the time to send a card. There are always psychological work-arounds, and you'll feel better if you find one.

- *Deal with your biases*—Perhaps you think that everyone past the age of eighty should move out of their apartment and into a facility for old people. If they don't, then you think they're taking unnecessary risks—and if they get hurt at home, or walking on the street alone, then it's their fault: "Why should I empathize with someone who won't do what's right?" Well, what's "right" in your opinion may not be in theirs. Maybe they're still entirely mobile, and they like being independent. If they fall or get hurt at home, they may have been more vulnerable than other people but still not *so* vulnerable that you shouldn't empathize. When you feel yourself withholding empathy, examine your biases and deal with them. Ask yourself, "Am I being unduly judgmental?" Most people deserve our empathy unless they've done something so awful as not to deserve it.

- *Listen attentively without interrupting*—Careful listening opens us up mentally and emotionally to another person. As we begin to *hear* them and process what they're saying, we'll start connecting what they say to our own experience. That's when empathy kicks in. While this is happening, don't interrupt with "solutions" that may just reflect your own biases or what you'd do in their position. What's right for you may not be right for them, and they may resent the suggestion—which could make you seem like you're not listening at all, but just trying to manage them. Listening attentively is about waiting until the person has had a chance to explain themselves fully. Then, try to get past your biases and offer constructive support.

- *Be curious*—Right now, you probably have a tight circle of friends. You get news from TikTok or other social media feeds programmed to reflect your interests. It's comfortable. But if you want to develop a greater awareness of the world—your place in it, its problems, the opportunities available to you—then you need to get outside your comfort zone. Read the newspaper. Meet people who are not just like you. Get involved with organizations that help people (okay, you're not ready to run them, but you can volunteer).

The point is to be exposed to people and situations that encourage you to understand the complexity of the world and of human relations. You want to become sensitized to things that are outside your immediate field of vision. You want to develop habits of thinking, and the skills to adequately respond, that you can draw on when the need for empathy arises.

- *Recognize that your emotions are like other people's—* Because we live in our own heads, we tend to think that our emotions are exclusively ours, rather than typical of the great mass of humanity. If you want to cultivate empathy, it's important to accept that while each person is unique, they experience the same range of emotions that you do. If something awful happens to them, they are likely to feel awful—just as you would. It's also important to recognize that at times, some people may experience a depth of emotion that's on a continuum with yours but even more intense. They may get clinically depressed, or anxious to the point where they can't cope (for example, they won't even go outside on a sunny day). The point is that if you see people are struggling, you can find it in yourself to relate to them.

- *You shouldn't try to be a substitute for professional help—* If you think they need help beyond what a friend or acquaintance can provide, then you might ask them, "Have you thought about talking with someone who deals with these kind of issues?" Don't just come right out and say, "You need help." Empathy requires tact.

You don't want to hurt someone even further with awkward offers of help.

While empathy is a natural impulse, it can further be developed as a skill. You can work on it. You can practice. When you read some story in the newspaper, maybe about some far-away disaster, ask yourself, "What would I say to the survivors? How would I make them feel that they're not forgotten?" The point is to be ready to empathize when you know that you should. It's also important to *know* that you should. Ask yourself, "Am I willing to expose myself by acknowledging that I know how they feel?" Don't just assume that it's nobody's business that you've felt sad in the past. You're no less a person in their eyes by acknowledging that you've lived a normal life. Nobody is ever an invulnerable cartoon figure.

What's important about teenagers building empathy?—You might still ask, "Why should I cultivate empathy now—can't I wait until I have more complex social and professional relationships?" The answer is that empathy can be a building block of morality, as well as an element of successful relationships in school and beyond. It can help you now to build connections that will last beyond school. It also helps you to develop helping behaviors that you'll need as you mature. The point is that it takes a long time to turn into the best version of ourselves. If we start when we're twenty or so, we might not get where we want to be until we're in our thirties—by which time we may have failed to sustain connections that we wish we still had. Along the way, we may feel awkward expressing empathy that comes easily to other people. Those people may become

135

team leaders before we do. They will have had more opportunities to feel better about themselves.

There has been substantial research into why empathy is important for teenagers' health and wellness. For example, empathy has been shown to prevent bullying and alleviate its effects. As everyone knows, teen bullying can be merciless. It is documented to have caused suicides among its more vulnerable victims. If teens felt more empathetic toward other teens, they would be less inclined to engage in bullying and better able to respond when someone they know is the victim of bullying.

Also, because teenagers' brains are still developing, a teen can lay down pathways that will stay with them as their brains continue to develop. This will provide an important defense against callousness, which—in some teens—is itself a defense against experiencing or becoming involved with other people's pain. In other words, empathy is a defense against undesirable, socially damaging traits that some teenagers mistakenly assume will help them survive in a chaotic world. Thus, while some teens live in an accidental cocoon, these teens live in a fortress of their own deliberate design. If they develop empathy, they'll be less inclined to want to stay there.

Some advocates even teach empathy to children in grade school. Roots of Empathy, for example, is an organization that helps children learn empathy by means of guided observations of an infant's development and emotions. The idea is to *accustom* children to empathy, so that it feels natural. The underlying assumption is that you can't start too early. If educators believe in starting with five- and six-year-olds, then it's probably not too early to begin thinking about empathy in your teens.

Empathy is not just one of those skills that it's nice to pick up when you can, like skiing. It's more like swimming, which can make a profound difference in your life. This is why educators are teaching it to children who can barely read. Try to commit to empathy. You'll find that the commitment pays off in terms of better relationships and enhanced professional success.

As an exercise, try to imagine a world where empathy has suddenly disappeared—it seems like an idea for a Stephen King novel. Things would start falling apart.

Takeaways—While the capacity for empathy is innate, there are mundane factors that can get in the way of expressing it. It's important to develop work-arounds, permitting you to be empathetic in situations where otherwise you would not be. You should start now, while your brain is still developing. It's possible to practice empathy, as you would any skill that you want to develop. It's worth the effort—research shows that when you're empathetic toward others, your happiness is enhanced.

Questions to ask yourself and to discuss:

- Do I understand the concept of empathy, and why it's important at my stage of life?
- Am I comfortable displaying empathy, or does it make me feel self-conscious?
- Have I considered how I could enhance my capacity for empathy?

- Do I know how to display empathy appropriately, depending on the situation and my relationship to the person with whom I empathize?
- Would I consider joining groups whose purpose is to show empathy to people unlike myself?
- As climate change increases, is it possible to feel empathy toward the planet, and is that what it will take to get real action from government and industry leaders?

Further reading

Friedberg, Ahron, MD, with Sandra Sherman. *Everyday Leadership: Taking Charge in the Real World.* Routledge, 2024.

King, Patrick. *Train Your Empathy: How to Cultivate the Single Most Important Relationship Skill.* Self published, 2022.

McLaren, Karla. *The Art of Empathy.* Sounds True, 2013.

Pfaff, Donald. *The Altruistic Brain: How We Are Naturally Good.* Oxford University Press, 2015.

Reiss, Helen, MD. *The Empathy Effect: Seven Neuroscience-based Keys for Transforming the Way We Live, Love, Work, and Connect Across Differences.* Sounds True, 2018.

Roots of Empathy, https://us.rootsofempathy.org/.

Chapter VIII

Building community helps you grow personally

We define ourselves in relation to others. We cultivate strong moral values because—whether we like it or not, though we should—we are actors in a drama whose thousands of other actors are affected by us and react to us. If we affect them in ways that they like, they'll react positively, and *we'll know it.* We'll keep acting that way because we like to be liked. After a while, our actions add up to a personality, which we recognize as our own. It happens to everyone. Such interactions, where we derive our sense of self (at least in part) from others' perceptions of us, is part of being human.

The same dynamic occurs when we display empathy.

But there's a wrinkle. Though we act in a world where, theoretically, lots of people see us, we really act in a far smaller sphere (except perhaps if we're the president, or someone of that stature). We act, and define ourselves, in a community, a relatively enclosed entity whose limited extent can be variously described, depending on its focus.

What is a community?—Here are some ways to conceptualize it.

- A group of people living in the same place (e.g., North Philly)
- A group having a particular characteristic in common (e.g., the scientific community)
- A feeling of fellowship with others, resulting from sharing common attitudes, interests, and goals (e.g., the sense of community that opposing nuclear proliferation can provide; alumni dedicated to supporting their alma mater)

A community results when people come together, formally or informally, because they have something (tangible or intangible) in common. This human convergence can be provisional, ad hoc, to meet a recently perceived need; it can also be that these people are the latest cohort in a long line of similarly situated people. Thus, a community is not just a geopolitical construction like, say, Great Neck, New York, which you can locate on a map. It *can* be, but it doesn't have to be.

You probably belong to several communities already. For example, your school is a community: everyone from the principal on down is in the same place, every day, and shares the same goal (they want the school to be a great place to learn). Parents may consider themselves an extended part of the community, and many of the alums may do so as well. As a student who's been there for some time, and who's grown comfortable on campus, you may consider the school your primary community ("That's where my friends are, and we all try to live by its 'pillars' of kindness, honor, purpose, and respect"). You identify with your school, and can't imagine who you'd be if you weren't there.

But now suppose that on weekends you work at a food co-op, offloading vegetables from a delivery truck, then making sure they're properly stored. The work is good exercise and fun; the people are your age and share your commitment to sustainable farming; you've gotten to know them through weekly meetings and by heading to Starbucks after work. From your perspective, the co-op is a community of maybe twenty workers, even though hundreds of people belong to the co-op, shop there, and support its mission. The people in your little community may not be your *best* friends (those are at school), but you like them, and you like sharing ideas about how to work more efficiently ("If the guys offloaded the biggest boxes, and the girls unpacked them, everything would go faster"). You like thinking of yourself as a co-op person, who's showing the wider community—the city where you live—that there's an eco-friendly alternative to the supermarket. Like your school, the co-op has shaped your sense of yourself.

As your membership in both communities demonstrates, they are not entirely exclusive of each other. In fact, several members of your school community belong to the co-op community (people in your class work there). It's natural for communities to intersect in this way, especially where there's some commonality in their defining features—here, for example, their members' ages and interests. But no matter what your classmates do, both communities intersect insofar as you're concerned, since you belong to both of them. You can think of "community" as one element in a Venn diagram that displays the various affiliations that help define you.

Of course, you're at the center. Your school, the co-op, and your other affiliations are the intersecting circles around you. These circles will shift (think of them as changing their color) as you drop out of one community and join another. The point is that throughout our lives, unless we live alone on a desert island, we are part of communities—some are more important to us than others, but we still belong to them. We may feel like we've outgrown them . . . but they're still in our head, if only as a persistent state of mind. For example, if you *ever* lived in North Philly, you remain part of that community, which has come to be defined not just by its location but by an indelible attitude ("Baby, you gotta have lived there to understand"). You recognize people from that community by how they act and what they say, even though neither of you may have lived there for years. If you do go back, you fall right into the old patterns—and revel in them.

We can be passive members of a community ("I never use my privileges at the country club"), or active ("I like working with rescue animals at the pound—I get a sense of belonging"). But even if a community does not define us very much ("I'm not from the Bronx as much as I used to be"), it's there. We sense it. It's the essence of community to provide not just a sphere of action but, in many cases, a way of looking at things (including ourselves). It can be a mental as well as a physical place, where—just by belonging—we feel part of something, as opposed to being strung out on our own. Maybe, when the need arises, we form an ad hoc community, which will meet the need and then quietly disband (for example, a local school needs new uniforms for the band, so some parents hold a bake sale). Still, once the need is met, the former members of the community think, "I couldn't have done that on my own." The idea of the community lingers and shapes our memories.

Organizations recognize the appeal of community. They know we want to feel part of something real, and full of people, when everything else seems so impersonal (have you seen those AI order-takers at fast food drive-thrus?), so when they ask you to donate blood, or patronize local businesses, they say "Help your community!" or "Your community needs you!" They conscript you into something larger than yourself because humans *like* to feel connected. We want the sense of belonging, support, friendship, purpose, and identity that community provides. Deep down, community is explained by neuroscience. North Philly (or its moral equivalent) is inextricably—and literally—in our heads because our *brains* evolved to ensure that we socialize. Alligators live solitary lives, but we don't. We survive and feel fully human in groups, especially where those groups confer some unique identity on us ("Baby, you gotta have lived there . . .").

The recent trend toward co-working environments demonstrates the appeal of communality. These environments tend to be large, open areas where people can plunk down with their computers but also walk around and meet other people. The idea is that this freedom promotes synergism—one geek talks to another, and the Next Big Thing takes off. Universities have discovered the idea as well. For example, Rockefeller University in New York City built a Collaborative Research Center, specifically designed to get scientists out of their labs and into spaces where they can share ideas without the formalities associated with presenting papers and publishing in peer-reviewed journals.

Of course, Facebook/Meta, TikTok, and an array of online platforms are full of communities, some highly specialized. For example, some are for lesbians who discover their sexual orientation later in life and need guidance on how to come out (for example, to husbands and children). These women report that it's comforting to know that other woman have faced similar issues and are there to provide support. For them, community is powerful—it gives them courage to start a new phase of their lives.

What does it mean to "build" a community, and why is it important to me?—Of course, you can just nominally belong to a community, the way scattered beekeepers, hand-carved furniture makers, or mountaineers might follow what's happening in their respective pursuits. Maybe you read a publication or go to an annual trade show. You might attend meetings of a local association and even pay dues. But while you've made friends over the years, and learned stuff, that's about all. The community is loosely organized, and your affiliation is tenuous. It would be a big change ("Hey, I like these guys, but we all mind our own business") if your bare-bones affiliation were kicked up a notch. You might even resist. Thus, for example, when the local beekeepers' group forms a committee to combat colony collapse disorder, you don't even think of joining. You know the committee is important (your own bees were suffering), but you don't feel like traveling to other cities and you figure someone else (whose bees are suffering more) will do it.

But from the perspective of your personal growth, you probably should have said yes.

Think about it. Had you made the commitment, you'd have helped build the beekeeping community both locally and across the country. Building a community means strengthening it; making it more cohesive and effective. Even if the community doesn't have a stated purpose—the way, for example, that co-working sites do—it has an unstated purpose of enabling its members to identify with each other in ways that bolster their identity *as members of the community*. If you identify as part of the queer community, your identity is firmer than if you were just you. You feel empowered by belonging. In the case of the beekeepers, the purpose was to keep raising bees in a sustainable environment. Therefore, to build that community, you'd work on behalf of its loosely articulated but still compelling purpose.

Perhaps you'd aggregate new USDA data on bees and share it with people who need it. You'd help to lobby governments to limit pesticides that are causing collapse. You'd draw beekeepers together to rally in support of an insect that pollinates 80 percent of our crops. As the committee's initiatives gain traction with the public, and the beekeeping community increases in clout, you will have contributed to something important—even beyond the community, because the country at large will reap the benefits. You will have grown personally as you became adept at pursuing the committee's work ("Hey, I'm actually good at explaining entomology to non-nerds").

The point is that when you contribute time and talent to a community and begin to define yourself in terms of those contributions, you grow into your work. You become more the person that you could be, if you just tried. Helping to build a community is the opposite of complacency, and thus the opposite of personal stagnation. It's work, but people are grateful, and you begin to appreciate what you can do if you make the effort. You learn about yourself. From a longer-term perspective, you develop skills and confidence that stay with you. You define yourself as a can-do person who overcomes obstacles ("The pesticide industry outspent us by orders of magnitude!") with determination and intelligence. You learn how to navigate within a group ("Some of those beekeepers were afraid to challenge government regulators for not doing enough, but I persuaded them") as well as externally. You may even become a leader.

Of course, it won't all happen at once. But commitment is just that—you stay with something. You build your capabilities, even as you help build the community.

Community-building also enhances your growth by exposing you to new people. You acquire soft skills. When (in the hypothetical scenario above) you visit beekeepers in other parts of the country, you talk with them, learn about their bees, and get a sense of the challenges they face (which likely vary with urban vs. rural environments). New people offer us new perspectives ("I stopped using neonicotinoids on my crops, and it made a huge difference") on how to talk with and what to tell other people. But beyond all this, it's always great to meet new people—there's a sense of discovery, and sometimes they become friends. You might visit them nonprofessionally if you're in their neighborhood. But you'll certainly become more sensitive to the nuanced behaviors that you encounter over a range of people. New people = personal growth.

In this regard, you'll also learn about group dynamics—the system of behaviors and psychological processes occurring within a group or between one group and another. Group dynamics is a huge field, touching everything from politics to leading a Girl Scout troop. It's crucial to managing a business and is taught in business schools. If you're helping to build a community—juggling internal and external relationships—you'll be observing and helping to orchestrate group dynamics (a fancy term for something you may not even have known you were engaged in). Think about that, and its implication for your next big act.

Getting bills through Congress is a feat of group dynamics (the Speaker of the House corrals a bunch of self-interested members to sign on to their party's policies). Novels are just one big imagined collection of group dynamics (George Eliot's *Middlemarch, A Study in Provincial Life*, written in 1871/2, is still the classic example, depicting relationships among people across generations in all social strata). The writers' strikes in Hollywood, which halted movie and TV production for months, were tugs-of-war in group dynamics that affected everyone—even those of us with no financial stake in the outcome. Whatever you're planning to do with your life, being up close and personal now, in an arena of group dynamics, will be hugely important to your personal growth.

Community-building, like empathy in the previous chapter, is a two-way street. Unlike in random assemblages of people, where you are largely anonymous, in a community you have an immediate identity ("She's one of us") that encourages people to support you and your work for the community. It's like in kinship theory in anthropology, where people tend to be most helpful to those with whom they have the greatest affinity. Parents help their own kids more than their sister's, and still more than their half-sister's. When you are doing something for the community—like helping to build its influence and resources—other members will feel strongly about helping *you*, professionally but also personally. You grow, professionally and personally, because so many other people (who share your concerns) want you to succeed. If you just keep on keeping on, their cumulative assistance will show in your performance. You'll learn the new stuff they (take pains to) show you.

While no community will always rubber-stamp what we want to do, it will be more inclined (because of the mutual affinity) to give us space and time to make our case. It will be less inclined to leave us feeling isolated, weird, and without resources. A community is a good place to seek personal growth, as opposed to seeking it on the outside. At the very least, it will cut us some slack because everyone understands the challenges. We don't have to explain ourselves—there's already a common denominator of shared concerns.

Then there are the intangibles. It's exciting to help build a community. It can be fun. When you see what you've accomplished, especially through the admiring eyes of others, you get a sense of yourself as an agent of change. You redefine yourself in ways that had not previously occurred to you. *You sense yourself growing*, like bamboo (it can shoot up three feet in a day). You also gain confidence that, perhaps, you can grow in new directions. You plausibly imagine what you might do ("I can help this community raise the funds it needs"), and then try to grow into the task. Community-building now is practice for your future.

It's important to find a community that you want to build. Figure out where you have the greatest affinity and could make an appropriate commitment. Maybe it's to your block association, which holds an annual kids' fair ("I could arrange for healthy snacks"). Maybe it's to the worldwide community that opposes diamond-mining practices that deprive workers of a living wage ("I could start a column in the school newspaper, raising my classmates' awareness"). It's up to you. But as you begin to act, you will grow for the reasons and in the ways that we've just discussed. In this sense, community-building is also like empathy in that what you feel is of little value to others unless you express it (and when you do express it, you benefit).

But suppose I want to get paid for what I do—why should I just volunteer?—You might say, "While everything about community-building sounds nice, as a teenager I'm not likely to get paid." That's a concern, especially with jobs available where you could earn real money (the minimum wage in Boston is $15/hour for non-tipped employees). You might even say, "I don't want to be a drudge, and sit around licking stamps." That's also a concern, since no one wants to be bored, or to put out effort just to learn nothing. But there's another way to approach these issues. There's a lot you can do that will allow you to be intellectually and emotionally engaged. If you choose the right activity—scouting for the Little League team or helping to coach it; helping a local food bank inspect donated groceries; teaching the flute in a group that serves inner-city kids—you're becoming part of a community and helping to build it. You'll feel good about yourself and kick-start your personal growth by meeting new people, getting more responsibility as people *see* what you can do, and laying the foundation for a great college application essay ("My Year Hunting for the Next Willie Mays").

If you can find a community whose work excites you; if you can do stuff you love; if they'll give you a chance to show what you can do; if you have a sense of belonging; and if they'll give you support, then you should consider making a commitment. Think of it as an investment of time and energy in your future. You don't think twice about investing time and energy at school. Helping to build a community offers some of the same paybacks.

How can I help build a community?—The previous discussion provides some examples, but you can multiply them endlessly. Here are some initial steps you can take before you make a commitment.

- *Choose a community*—Though you may be part of several communities already (your school, a place of worship, classical embroidery enthusiasts), look around—inside and outside your affiliations—before choosing one (or two at most, since you're busy with school) that you'd like to help build. Ask yourself, as well as people inside and outside the community, whether a community shares your values, whether it will offer you support, and whether the people are friendly (or too busy to pay you much attention). Find out whether your personal style is compatible with theirs (maybe you're an activist, while they prefer subtlety and non-confrontation).

Find out about communities that do the kind of work you'd like to be involved in *over time* (commitments take time, and building anything is a process). Talk to people who may know more about the general area than you do. In other words, don't commit yourself until you find a community where you'll be comfortable, and to which you'd like to contribute now and into the future—not forever, but long enough so you'll feel you've accomplished something.

It's not a good idea to casually shop around, trying out one community and then another. Of course, even after some conscientious investigation, you may discover that you've made a mistake—you don't like the people, or no one gives you any responsibility. But most of the time, you can avoid this type of situation by talking with people you'll be working with and asking them honest questions.

- *Determine how you can contribute, and whether the community could use (and be receptive to) what you can do*—Various communities will be interested in some of your skills and not others. The food bank, for example, won't care about your uncanny ability to steal bases. But if you think you have something to contribute, then try to find out if they'd be interested. You may excel in some area that's in line with what they do, but they may already have enough people doing it ("We don't need any more flute teachers, but if you can teach the trombone . . .").

- *Decide what you hope to get out of the experience, and whether you can get it from a particular community*—Book clubs, social justice communities, and environmental groups may all offer different experiences. The book club may ask you to attract new, younger readers; the environmental group may want you to be another pair of eyes and ears, locating violations of dumping and noise regulations. You'll learn something either way, but maybe you'd rather strengthen an organization that's concerned with local health. In that case, go for the latter.

- *Find role models*—Perhaps you know or know of people who have helped to build a community. It doesn't have to be a leader, but just someone whose work has contributed to progress in a community.

- *Be open to new experiences*—Even though you may want to design your community-building experience, you should still be open to new experiences and new sorts of people that you haven't yet thought of. Feeling comfortable is important, but so is the chance to learn stuff that's off your personal radar. If you discover some opportunity that seems unlike anything you've already thought of, don't just dismiss it. Think about. Talk to people. Find out more.

- *Give yourself enough time*—You don't need to rush into anything. If you'd like to devote the summer to community-building, start investigating several months in advance. Put all your data together before making any decisions. It's a serious decision, and it should be as close to the right one as you can make it.

- *Start a community on your own*—If you have a great idea (a nonprofit that enlists people to build bird sanctuaries in their yards?), and you think you can build a community around it, then perhaps you could give it a try. You might have to raise funds, build a website, and do the publicity, but that's all part of your personal growth. Maybe get help from a few of your friends. Maybe keep a journal. It's worth a shot.

While you benefit from becoming part of a community, it's important to find your niche. In Chapter VI, this *Guide* discussed the challenges of forming healthy relationships. Finding a community that you want to help build can be just as challenging, usually for the same reasons—Do I get along with the people? Do I feel generous toward them? Do they feel that way toward me? How will I feel down the road? Before making a commitment, perform what's called due diligence. In business, this means that you take all reasonable steps to appraise a deal before entering into it. You may feel passionate about a community, but there's no need to act impetuously before you start helping to build it.

When you choose, and start helping to build a community, you'll learn that not everything turns out how you think it will. A community—especially one that's been around for a while—has a life of its own. But if you join it, then do so with a generosity of spirit, and don't expect an immediate payoff. Don't even expect a tangible payoff ("Hey, when I worked for the food bank, I learned how to grade produce—this could lead to a *real* job next year"). If your confidence and self-esteem increase, and if you've learned how to get along with lots of new people, then you've made a contribution to your personal growth.

You will also have joined a rapidly growing movement. Community-building is everywhere—just look at the slew of how-to books on Amazon (we've listed just a few below). Maybe that's because people are tired of government squabbling and want to be directly involved in projects close to home that affect their lives. These people are experimenting. They're dreaming up new approaches to both old and new problems. Maybe this is a vision of the future. You could be a part of it.

Takeaways—While community-building may take time, you should consider it an investment in your personal growth. But it's important to perform due diligence before you choose a community where you want to become involved. Remember, making a commitment is serious, and you should be prepared to follow through. Once you do, however, you will meet new people, learn about group dynamics, and gain valuable experience. Your self-confidence will tick upward. You'll feel good about doing good.

Questions to ask yourself and to discuss:

- What communities do I belong to, and which ones do I think I might like to join?
- Am I prepared to adequately investigate communities that interest me, and what qualities would I want to find in them?
- How would I like to help build a community? What values would I like to advance?
- What skills do I have to offer a community, and which ones would I like to develop?
- Do I have community-building role models?
- Am I interested in forming a new community, and do I have skills and resources to do it?

Further reading

Eliot, George. *Middlemarch: A Study in Provincial Life.* Penguin Classics, 1871–1872.

Friedberg, Ahron, MD, with Sandra Sherman. *Everyday Leadership: Taking Charge in the Real World.* Routledge, 2024.

Gruber, James. *Building Community: Twelve Principles for a Healthy Future.* New Society Publishers, 2020.

Kyte, Richard. *Finding Your Third Place: Building Happier Communities (and Making Friends Along the Way).* Fulcrum, 2024.

Minkler, Meredith, et al. *Community Organizing and Community Building for Health and Equity.* Rutgers University Press, 2021.

Stanley, Andy, and Bill Willits. *Creating Community: Five Keys to Building a Thriving Small Group Culture.* Multnomah, 2021.

Studer, Quint. *Building a Vibrant Community: How Citizen-Powered Change is Reshaping America.* Be the Bulb, 2023.

Chapter IX

Nurturing a sound mind is important to physical health

Your feelings—your inner life—profoundly affect your physicality. You can't function at your peak if you're anxious, depressed, or suffering from post-traumatic stress disorder (PTSD). If you're distracted by any of these, or even just by irrational fears (do you *hate* crowds, or airplanes, or getting a shot in your arm?), you'll forget to eat right. You might break out in hives. Maybe you'll skip the dentist because you'd rather have a toothache than submit to novocaine. Of course, there are millions of reasons why you may become upset. The point is to recognize and deal with them. This chapter—like the others—involves being honest with yourself. You need to acknowledge what may be going on (or going wrong) in your head. Then you can begin to address what needs to be fixed. It's not enough to say "Oh, that's just me," if you're slowed down or even disabled by a chronic psychological condition. In those situations, the better response is: "My psychology and physical well-being seem out of sync, so I'll find out why and get back on track."

Sometimes you may not even know, precisely, how to identify a psychological problem—you may just feel vaguely distracted, bored, or out of sorts. It's okay not to be an expert. You can get help. But if you do have a problem, don't ignore it. Psychological problems usually don't go away on their own. They require intervention—first by you and then, if necessary, by a professional. If you start with the premise that the choices you make now will affect your future, then you'll address adverse psychological conditions that could keep you from being (and becoming) the best version of yourself.

The mind/body connection is profound. It's simply not possible to say, "I'm anxious/stressed/depressed, but if I don't fall asleep in class I don't have *real* problems." Psychological problems are just as real as physical ones, and they can become physical at any time. In fact, if you have certain persistent physical problems (like falling asleep in class), this could be a sign of psychological issues that need attention. Especially in otherwise healthy young people, the two often go together. Thus, it's crucial that you think of yourself as one organism, whose psychological and physical components constitute You. In biology class, you wouldn't say that your brain is somehow separate from the rest of you, so when you reflect on yourself as you go through the day, you can't say, "I just don't let my feelings affect the rest of my life." There's no such thing as "the rest," since you're *all* you. The same areas of your brain through which you experience emotion also light up from pain.

Yet, even if you're aware that psychological problems are affecting your performance, you may not want to rock someone else's boat by talking about yourself.

Young people tend not to share painful or difficult feelings, especially with their parents, whom they want to protect. But it's important that you get past any self-consciousness in this regard. When there were public safety crises on the streets of several major cities, signs went up pleading, "If you see something, say something" (the plea is now a national campaign). Think about that if you sense something in yourself that is troubling and even bewildering in terms of how you might deal with it. The whole point of saying something is that you don't have to know what to do—experts are there to help, provided that you alert them.

This chapter is not meant to frighten you ("Am I screwed up and don't even know it?"). But it is intended to make you aware of how your mind and body interact, so that psychological problems can *become* physically manifest. They can diminish your performance across an array of parameters, from whether you eat right to whether you can concentrate at school.

But is all this still theoretical ("Don't look at *me*, I don't have issues")? Absolutely not! Vast numbers of teenagers turn to recreational drugs to alleviate anxiety about even routine parts of everyday life—like navigating the demands of family or choosing the right outfit. They're irritable; extremely sensitive to criticism; they avoid new and difficult situations; they repeatedly seek reassurance. They feel pressure to be perfect and beat themselves up when they can't be. Since so much of their life revolves around school (academics, sports, socializing), their performance at school (or lack of it) can pre-cipitate anxiety/stress/depression. They stay home; they do as little as possible to get by; they can't even think about college, which just seems like a bigger, scarier version of what they're already experiencing.

In 2024, the surgeon general argued that social media should carry warnings about its potential threat to adolescent mental health. Since you and your friends use social media every day, you're all potentially at risk. Again, concerns about your mental health are not theoretical. Think about it. If you follow people whose lives seem more interesting than yours ("I shouldn't look at their posts, but I can't help it"), or whose bodies seem more toned ("I'm at the gym every day, but so what?") you can see how its allure can also drive you nuts.

What does a sound mind look like?—Sometimes we go through the day and feel like different people from one hour to the next ("I barely know myself before breakfast!"). How is it possible to tell what a sound mind really is? Well, there are cer-tain basic qualities that stay with us, no matter how we feel from one hour (or day, or week) to the next. Primarily, these qualities revolve around the concept of resilience, discussed in Chapter III. If you're able to bounce back from disappointments ("I didn't make the swim team, but next semester I'll try out for soccer"), then you won't fall into some trough of self-fulfilling grief ("If I'm such a crummy swimmer, they probably won't want me on any team"). You won't predispose yourself to stress and anxiety.

Another quality of a sound mind is the ability to shift your perspective so that you don't become rigid. If something doesn't work, you try something else. You don't write yourself off as a failure. Rather, you adjust your aspirations and keep on going. You accept that life is rarely linear. You go with the flow. You overcome the resistance posed by your own prejudices. You bounce ideas off family and friends, and you draw on their support. You're not afraid to open yourself up to people, and you listen to them when they talk.

So, you don't just have a sound mind—you cultivate it. You take care of yourself by maintaining a healthy diet, exercising, and finding time to reflect. When you find yourself facing a challenge, you don't panic. Instead, you call on your personal resources and ask, "What can I do to get past it?" When something isn't going your way, you don't take your marbles and go home. Instead, you ask, "What else is out there, and how can I make the most of it?" Having a sound mind means *actively* having a sound mind. Like most things, it's work.

Of course, sometimes nothing works. You don't feel right. At that point, it's up to you to recognize the signs that you may have issues, and then deal with those issues effectively.

What does psychological trouble look like?—Everybody thinks they're a little weird ("I always comb my hair the second I get up," "I don't eat canned foods—there's one chance in a billion of botulism"). Most of the time, our quirks make us interesting. But sometimes what occurs in our head can have consequences that damage our well-being. Here are some problems to look out for. You'll notice some overlap among them, which is why their treatments (when we discuss them) will display some overlap as well.

Stress—Stress is a normal response to physical, emotional, and intellectual demands. It manifests as a type of strain or tension ("I'm at my limit, and pushing right past it!"). For example, when you move to a new community, meet new people, take an important test, or run a 10K, you may experience stress. But that's not always bad. While a temporarily elevated stress level produces anxiety ("Do I have the guts to pull this off?"), you may be spurred to work harder—and, finally, succeed. Such stress is adaptive and can leave you feeling stronger. However, when people say they "feel stressed," they tend to mean that their usual ways of coping with stress—walking a mile, watching TV—aren't working. Their stress level keeps rising, and it stays elevated. *They will experience many of the same symptoms listed above regarding the effects of anxiety, as well as some others.* For example:

- People under stress may be more accident-prone, since they are distracted and lack the necessary focus.
- Their blood pressure will go up; they'll experience heart palpitations; they can become breathless.
- Their muscles will feel tight.
- They'll grind their teeth while they sleep.
- They'll lose confidence and experience a sense of dissatisfaction ("I'm so stressed that I can't follow through with my vacation plans—and maybe I don't want to anyway").

Stress can lead to a vicious cycle of self-defeating actions (or non-actions and paralysis). It frequently results in increased use of drugs, tobacco, and alcohol. Later, this chapter will discuss how to manage stress.

Anxiety disorders and related conditions—These include excessive nervousness, fear, and worry. Of course, it's normal to feel some level of anxiety when our safety, health, or happiness is threatened. But when anxiety is disproportional to the threat, when it persists beyond the threat, or when it's overwhelming, then there's a problem.

Some common anxieties:

- **Generalized anxiety disorder** (GAD), excessive, persistent, unrealistic worry about everyday things. Such worries may appear for no apparent reason and can cause feelings of being constantly overwhelmed, fear, and apprehension.
- **Social anxiety disorder**, fear of being embarrassed or rejected in social situations.
- **Hypochondria**, or excessive worry about your health ("I hurt my hand playing football—now it will get infected and I'll get gangrene and it will have to be amputated").
- **Sudden panic attacks** ("I don't remember my lines, and the play starts in ten minutes!").
- **Fear of crowds**, or of finding yourself in large open spaces.
- **Body-type anxiety**, which can result in anorexia, bulimia, or a type of morbid self-hate ("I'm ugly and unattractive and my hair is stringy").
- **Post-Traumatic Stress Disorder (PTSD)**, which can result after traumatic events like rape or a car

accident—if something reminds you of the trauma, you can become depressed or frightened.

- **Obsessive Compulsive Disorder (OCD)**, where you can't control your thoughts, and can't seem to let go of things ("Will my cat eat the goldfish when I'm out for the day?").

If you have an anxiety disorder, these are some of the possible physical effects.

- **Restlessness**, feeling on edge, an inability to relax— you can't sit still
- **Difficulty controlling your emotions**, leading to outbursts ("Once I start worrying, I lash out at people; I scream; I blame everyone who's near me— especially those who are trying to help.")
- **Mood swings**, feelings of detachment—neither you nor anyone can predict whether you'll be withdrawn or outgoing
- **Trouble concentrating or focusing**—you're doing too many things and none of them well
- **Increased heart rate**, chest pains, dizziness, trembling
- **Hives and rashes**—conditions like psoriasis and eczema can be exacerbated
- **Insomnia**
- **Headaches**, body aches
- **Digestive issues**, including diarrhea and nausea
- **Feeling out of control** ("If I get behind the wheel, I'll break the speed limit and cause an accident.")

Obviously, anxiety can have stark physical consequences. It can affect the people around you. But it's treatable. The point is to find the right treatment, and not keep it bottled up. You may not even be *able* to keep it bottled up, since people will notice your mood swings, your lack of focus, or if you seem out of control. Later, this chapter will discuss ways to deal with anxiety.

Depression—Stress and anxiety can lead to depression, though it has several other causes as well. We all feel depressed occasionally, especially since the term is used loosely to cover a variety of blahs. But here are some symptoms that should concern you if you can't seem to shake them.

- **Persistent sadness**—you feel hopeless, to the point where even minor obstacles seem like huge obstacles
- **Low self-esteem**, extreme dislike for yourself
- **Loss of interest** in most activities and in personal relationships
- **Inability to socially interact**—you may be irritable and withdrawn, turn silent, and avoid people
- **Loss of energy, fatigue**—this can feel like it has a physical cause ("Oh, my muscles just aren't working"), but it can also reflect your loss of interest in things and low self-esteem ("I won't accomplish anything anyway, so why bother?")
- **Abnormal sleep patterns**
- **A change in appetite** that can lead to rapid weight gain or loss
- **Suicidal thoughts**, reckless behavior

Like anxiety and stress, depression has real physical effects. Nor does it usually go away on its own, especially if the underlying causes—a bad relationship, family strife, smoking—persist. We might not even think of some causes. For example, the link between social media and depression, especially around body image and social success, is increasingly apparent (even though addicted users think it makes them happy). Just the need to make hard choices can throw some people into depression.

Later, this chapter will examine ways to deal with depression. But it's up to you to think about (a) whether you have a problem, and (b) who might be a good person with whom to talk it over. You are responsible for your own well-being— before involving anyone else. Take time to reflect every day (see Chapter IV). Slow down and ask yourself, "How do I feel? How would I describe my feelings to someone else?" Make such queries a habit. You can't tell other people about your feelings if you can't find words for them.

How can I deal with anxiety, stress, and depression?

It's possible to have more than one of these conditions at once. For example, constant stress can lead to depression. You might experience undifferentiated symptoms that, together, leave you somewhere on the blah spectrum. But because these symptoms may run together, recommendations for dealing with one may be effective in dealing with another ("I thought I was trying to relieve my stress, but now my depression has lifted!"). It happens all the time.

Of course, the best way to deal with troubling psychological conditions (whatever they're technically called) is to prevent them. That's part of what nurturing a sound mind means. For example:

- If you're in a relationship where you feel used or abused, then find someone else (see Chapter VI).
- As you plan your future, don't rush into choices that you'll regret—this applies to near- and long-term plans.
- Don't smoke/drink/take drugs (which are ineffective coping mechanisms), and don't disappear into social media at the expense of friendships.
- Get enough sleep and eat a healthy diet.
- Spend time every day in self-reflection and cultivate self-awareness.

You don't need elaborate self-care regimens that are mostly celebrity-driven and tend to be one-size-fits-all. If you take the sensible steps cited above, and if you adopt habits that promote resilience, you'll be much better off. But if you sense that something isn't right, don't just let things slide.

Apart from steps you can take to try to prevent troubling psychological conditions, there are ways to deal with them if they occur. In the discussion below, you'll notice that what applies to anxiety may also be effective against stress and depression. You'll also notice that what may be useful in preventing adverse psychological conditions may also be useful—to a degree—in alleviating these conditions or reducing their severity. There's a continuum between prevention and alleviation; some steps will work sometimes; other steps will work at other times; some may not work at all or may just be partially effective. Everyone reacts differently. Don't expect miracles, though you can some-times expect to be surprised. Finally, don't expect any of these recommendations to be instantly effective. Some people react more quickly than others, so give yourself a chance to adjust to a new, potentially more beneficial regime:

Dealing with anxiety, stress, and depression—Many of these will sound like common sense, but that's because they've been shown to work. You don't have to deploy all of them, so choose some that seem likely to work for you.

- *Combat loneliness*—One of the best ways to deal with anxiety is to reduce your isolation. If you've become withdrawn, then find people and activities that you like. In fact, research demonstrates that getting involved in helping other people—maybe even just by listening—can make you feel better. You feel more valuable. Your self-esteem increases.
- *Appreciate the present*—Pay attention to what's happening around you right now, rather than dwelling on the past or staring down an imponderable future. Take everything a moment at a time, and try to see its value. In other words, practice mindfulness (see Chapter III).
- *Exercise*—Take exercise breaks. Try yoga. Go for a walk. Any of these can be combined with combating loneliness or (at the opposite extreme) making time for mindfulness or self-reflection.
- *Manage your time*—Anxiety frequently arises because you haven't left enough time. So plan your day or

your week so that you have enough time to do what you have to. Keeping a checklist also helps.

- *Turn it off!* —If your environment is a multi-decibel cacophony, turn down the music. If social media is making you feel inadequate, disconnect. The point is to distance yourself from or at least reduce the effect of distracting, aggravating stimuli. Anxiety gets worse when you're overstimulated or agitated.

- *Start a journal*—Good old-fashioned writing slows you down and forces you to think. It helps you put your concerns in perspective ("Okay, I guess I can try to . . . which I haven't done yet"), and to find work-arounds that you haven't thought of until you had to think. You might even discover you're a born storyteller.

- *Stop imagining the worst*—If you're making a presentation the next day, stop thinking about all the things that could go wrong ("I could lose my place," "The PowerPoint will seem blurry"). You could talk yourself into a kind of hysteria. Instead, imagine how great you'll feel when people applaud. You're a lot less fallible—and a whole lot smarter—than you dare to think you are.

- *Laugh at yourself*—We are all tiny dots in an infinite universe. Put your life in perspective. Establish a little distance from yourself, as you would if you were looking at a pointillist painting. If you're less wrapped up in yourself, and more engaged with everyone else, you'll feel less stressed.

- *Create a routine*—Routines, like exercising before dinner and cleaning up afterward, are coping mechanisms. Your life seems less scattered. You feel more in control, less vulnerable to anxieties and stressors that can lead to depression.
- *Stay connected, keep busy*—Depression tends to become entrenched when you don't have enough to do to occupy your mind. Stay connected with friends and pursue hobbies.
- *Consider mindfulness*—Chapter III examines mindfulness. You can use it any time to remain in the moment and detach yourself from what's making you depressed.

Of course, you may want to talk with a therapist about managing your condition. If you have severe physical symptoms, like a continually racing heart, then you should talk with a physician who can treat such conditions. In fact, you may want to seek help even while you're trying to help yourself—the two are hardly exclusive. Listen to your body and pay attention to the mind/body interface. You don't want your condition to become even worse.

Many young people respond well to cognitive behavioral therapy (CBT), which offers them strategies for thinking differently about anxiety, and for dealing with it when it occurs. On its website, the Child Mind Institute states: "By tolerating anxiety rather than avoiding things that trigger it, [teenagers] learn that it diminishes over time. And by gradually increasing exposure to feared objects or activities (a type of CBT called exposure therapy), the anxious response itself is reduced or eliminated." For example, if you're so afraid of public speaking that you break out in hives, CBT will gradually accustom you to making presentations. Eventually, your anxiety reaction will diminish or even disappear.

There are also medications, which you should only take under a licensed therapist's supervision. But the point is that help is available. You need enough presence of mind to determine when to seek it.

If you ever feel desperate, the Suicide and Crisis Hotline number is **988**. A real human being will be there for you, 24/7, every day of the year.

Your mind and body are profoundly connected. Your feelings affect your physicality (the reverse is also true; sickness can easily make you anxious/stressed/depressed). You need to be attentive to how, in your own case, this mind/body connection is manifest ("Does my anxiety affect my sleep?" "Is stress causing my heart to race?"). Of course, you may not know just what's troubling you, or how some clinician would identify it. Nonetheless, if you feel that your feelings are vague but real and troubling, that's reason enough to seek help. The point is to get back into gear and become the best version of yourself—now and into the future.

Takeaways—The mind/body connection is profound. Adverse psychological conditions such as anxiety, stress, and depression can lead to adverse physical conditions that, if not addressed,

(Continued . . .)

can undermine your ability to be the best version of yourself. It's important to be attentive to changes in your feelings, and to take corrective steps if you know that they're not what you're accustomed to. Even if your feelings have not yet physically slowed you down, they can. Help is always available if you need it. You can help yourself by becoming more resilient and opening up your perspective.

Questions to ask yourself and to discuss:

- Do I understand the symptoms of anxiety, stress, and depression?
- Have I developed habits that will help me from becoming overly anxious, stressed, or depressed, or do my habits have the opposite effect?
- Am I willing to share my feelings with people that I trust, or am I embarrassed or afraid to be open?
- Do I regularly reflect on myself, or am I so busy that I don't take time to understand my feelings?
- If I notice physical symptoms such as insomnia or loss of appetite, do I think about whether they could have a psychological cause?
- After reading this *Guide*, do I now have a more holistic view of myself, and do I recognize how the mind and body function together?

Further reading

Banks, Richard. *How to Deal with Stress, Depression, and Anxiety: A Vital Guide on How to Deal with Nerves and Coping with Stress, Pain, OCD, and Trauma.* Next Level International, 2021.

Child Mind Institute. "Guide to Behavioral Treatments." https://childmind.org/guide/guide-to-behavioral-treatments/.

Friedberg, Ahron, MD, with Sandra Sherman. *Life Studies in Psychoanalysis: Faces of Love.* Routledge, 2023.

Halloran, Janine. *Coping Skills for Teens: 60 Helpful Ways to Deal with Stress, Anxiety, and Anger.* Encourage Play, 2021.

Johnson, Shawn. *Attacking Anxiety: From Panicked and Depressed to Alive and Free.* Thomas Nelson, 2022.

Meurisse, Thibaut. *Master Your Emotions: A Practical Guide to Overcome Negativity and Better Manage Your Feelings.* Self published, 2018.

Trenton, Nick. *Stop Overthinking: 23 Techniques to Relive Stress, Stop Negative Spirals, Declutter Your Mind, and Focus on the Present.* Self published, 2021.

Chapter X

Making the most of good choices leads to a fulfilling life

Chapter I discussed how to make good choices—take your time, consider the options, measure the risks. Now let's assume you've made some, like staying fit and finding the right group of friends. Can you just sit back and relax? Of course not. Making good choices is the *first step* in a long-term maintenance regimen, where you follow up by taking important actions that give your choices continuing effect, even as circumstances change. If you chose to stay fit, you work out every day and eat nutrient-dense food. You play tennis. You walk a mile instead of taking the bus. If you've found good friends, you cultivate them. You pay attention to *their* lives and support them when they need you. In other words, you act positively to make your choices effective. You remain fit, even though schoolwork is challenging. You keep your friends, rather than letting them drift away. You don't let things go by default. You're committed to being—and becoming—the best version of yourself.

Making the most of good choices involves *living* your good habits—Think back to Chapter II, which discussed conscious eating. You choose the right foods, in the right balance for your body type. After a while, these choices ("Should I go for ice cream or a peach?") stop being one-time mega-decisions that you ponder every time the dessert tray rolls around. Rather, you allow them to become habits. They become integral to how you eat—all the time, every day, except perhaps in special circumstances (where you deviate as little as possible, then bounce back to your personal norm). Choosing the less caloric option on a regular basis is your way of making the most of an initial choice to eat well.

Good-choices-turned-habits allow us to make the most of those choices without having to go back to square one every time. We're on a trajectory of follow-throughs. So, while we might not always choose fruit for dessert—we might take a cookie—we'll still be acting *within parameters* that allow us keep making the most of our initial good choice. No Oreos!

If you apply this principle to your whole life, and keep following through once you've made good choices, your life will be the product of all your good choices, instead of just a series of one-time resolutions that don't add up to much. You'll still have variety in your life (so many different fruits! so many different cookies!), but you'll have passed up options that are inconsistent with your initial good choice.

When you make the most of good choices (allowing them to become habits), you're extending the present into the future, which can present challenges that (but for the habit) would give you an excuse to slack off. For example, if you've made a habit of keeping in touch with friends, you'll stay in touch even when they've gone to a different college. Maybe you'll see them over the holidays, even though it's harder because your family moved to the suburbs when you graduated ("Oh, I'll have to take a train—but it's worth it to keep up"). Even though circumstances have changed, you're still following through. You compensate for those changes. In effect, *making the most of a good choice starts one second after you've made that choice.* It's about designing and then building your life into what you'd like it to be. If you need to adapt, you do.

Ideally, once your choices become habits, following through is relatively easy. But when it's not so easy, as with your friend who's now farther away, you still find the means to make the most of your choice. Life is full of obstacles to being and becoming our best selves, but making the most of good choices means that you find a way to get past those obstacles.

Part of the reward is that there is often a synergy between making the most of one choice and making the most of another. For example, if you've followed through on your choice to eat well, you're better positioned to keep fit. Our choices, and the habits that reinforce them as we mature, begin to fill in the contours of our life with actual substance. Our choices segue from isolated events ("Oh, today I chose to eat right") into the matrix of activities that constitute whom we have chosen to be ("I'm someone who always eats right and stays fit"). We may not be exactly the person we want to be, but we've tried to get as close as we can.

You can think of this process—this becoming—as what happens when we look at a pointillist painting. Up close, it looks like a lot of smalls dots, but as we stand back, the image emerges. Our eyes allow us to fill in the spaces and see the image as the artist intended.

This chapter is all about process. How do I make the most of my good choices? How do I keep on keeping on despite the inevitable challenges? How do I build a life that reflects the cumulative effect of my good choices (even if I'm not exactly whom I set out to be)? In this sense, this chapter is related to Chapter III, which is about adopting good habits despite all the excuses we might make because, in the moment, they're an easy out when we face the work of doing what's right. The point is to get past the challenges—and the easy excuses—so that we can live our best lives.

We want to live our best lives in many dimensions. We want to keep fit. We want to eat well. We need to maintain our friendships. You could add to the list, based on what matters to you ("I want to be a success in business," "I want to be a professional dancer"). Getting to any such place, let alone several, requires us to develop strong habits. Along the way, we may have to sacrifice some dimension of our lives so that we can focus on others—there's that old saying at Oxford that you can socialize, be a scholar, and be an athlete, just not all at once. Our goals change. We grow. Sometimes something has to give. It's just that we should always working toward and live in ways that add up to some version of fulfillment.

We want to be happy with our choices, and not backtrack or regret or feel paralyzed. Ask yourself, "Did I give that choice a fair chance before I rejected it?" After all, while a choice is only good if it works for you, you can't blame the *choice* if you didn't *try* to make it work. Of course, in hindsight, a choice that seemed good when you made it may turn out to have been suboptimal ("I thought I should be a lawyer, but it turns out I should have been a doctor"). At that point you may want to go in a different direction, provided it's possible—which it isn't always. Circumstances may not allow you to, and besides, life isn't infinite. But even if you made a suboptimal choice, you may still be able to find ways of making the most of it ("I chose a geekier college than I should have, but I joined the drama club and I'm loving it"). Making the most of a choice starts from where we are now. In effect, you're running the process in reverse, repairing choices by finding new ways to make the most of them.

What is a fulfilling life?—You might say, "I'm following through on choices that seem to have been pretty good, but how do I know if I'm fulfilled? If I'm happy most of the time, is that enough?" Of course, there is no simple answer. Everyone's life is different. But here are a few common indicators of fulfillment against which to measure your own life:

- *A life that is meaningful and purposeful, and that aligns with your values and dreams*—Perhaps you choose to become a professional dancer, and ultimately to found a dance company that will bridge the gap between eastern and western dance forms and the cultures that they represent. You practice eight hours a day, attract patrons, and finally found a company that toured the world. When interviewed, you say, "My values are all about world peace, and I dreamed of becoming part of the peace process, helping cultures that disliked each other to appreciate each other." This work gives purpose to your life. You feel as though your life means something because you are changing people's suspicions of each other into admiration.

Maybe you choose to study linguistics and, after earning a PhD, you decide to create a program that allows humans to interpret the complex sounds of other mammals—such as dolphins and whales—and "talk" to them about avoiding parts of their habitat that are warming faster than others. You apply for a grant, explaining, "If we can communicate with other mammals in their own language, then we can help to save them from climate change." The grantor agrees, and allows you $1 million in start-up funds. Your life has a purpose. It aligns with your values. You think that that long slog through graduate school was finally worth it.

- *You feel energized, alive, at the top of your game—you know you're making an impact*—Suppose you work at a drug company, investigating new drugs that can inexpensively treat tropical diseases like Lassa fever, which often causes fatal hemorrhages. You and your team are achieving encouraging results. When you talk among yourselves, everyone agrees that they entered the field to make a difference in people's lives. You love the camaraderie; you feel energized; you feel vindicated for having studied biology rather than business (like everyone else in your family). When your mother calls, you tell her, "I made the right choice, and I could do this ten hours a day—I know it will pay off in lives saved." You can't imagine doing anything else.

Or you volunteer at a food bank and think it should work with local farms to bring fresh produce to inner-city kids. But when you join the management committee, everyone says, "We've always collected leftovers from restaurants—that's our model." You think they resent you for trying to shake things up. So you talk with other volunteers, who like your idea. You talk with local farms, who are eager to show they don't just sell fancy produce to high-priced restaurants. You draw up a plan, demonstrating how the food bank could radically improve kids' diets. You go on local talk radio to promote your idea. Finally, when management realizes how complacent they seem, they give the go-ahead to put your plan into action. When talk radio asks for another interview, you tell them, "I saw the chance to help kids, but I knew I'd face opposition. I figured out how to get past it, and now I'm making an impact on kids' health." You've made the most of a good choice.

- *You've achieved your goal in your career, relationship, or family life*—Maybe you wanted to become a partner in a Wall Street law firm. You worked hard at law school, kept your head down for eight years, played

the game when you had to . . . and then, wow, you
made it! You can hardly believe your luck, except
that you know that luck was barely a part of your
achievement. You did everything right. If you feel
fulfilled, it's because you *didn't* trust to luck. You tell
younger associates, "Look, I made choices. They're not
for everyone, but I worked at them and they worked
for me." Now you're where you wanted to be.

The same principle applies to a relationship, or
to your family. You finally married the person you
fantasized about for years ("Will they even look at
me?"). Now you've got adorable kids and, at least
emotionally, your life seems great. You tell your
friends, "I really value sharing my life on an intimate,
loving basis, and now it's worked out just as I'd
hoped." It's not easy bringing up kids, but when you
see how beautifully they're developing—and you
realize how much of the burden your spouse shares—
you couldn't be happier.

- *You've got great friends and activities that you enjoy*—
You love hanging out with your friends and going on
hikes with them. You love the bridge club that you
joined ("Everyone wants me for their partner"). You
love cooking, going to cooking classes, and sharing
the homemade breads and preserves that have become
your specialty. If people ask, you tell them, "Okay, I'm
single and my career is in the rear-view mirror. But
I feel fulfilled because I have great friends, and I've
never been so creative!" You got to this place through

a different kind of effort than the guy who made partner, but it *was* an effort and you're proud of it. You worked at making friends, just as you worked at learning how to cook. Now you can fill your days with people and activities that make you feel great.

Fulfillment takes different forms in each of these cases, but there's a common denominator: each person made good choices (or, rather, good choices within *their* frame of reference) and followed through sufficiently to make the most of those choices. The lawyer is a partner, the biology student is finding life-saving drugs. While there is no one-size-fits-all formula for feeling fulfilled, we all need follow-through regimens that help us make the most of our choices. When, for example, the lawyer had to work alongside colleagues whom he disliked, did he just throw in the towel and go home? Of course not. He figured out how to get assigned cases that his colleague wasn't on. To him, following through meant developing a plausible work-around. His favorite joke was, "Hey, a work-around is still work. I'm still doing my best."

In fact, developing contingency plans is part of any follow-through regime. You decide *in advance* that if this zig occurs, you'll zag in a different direction and still get where you're going. Planning for contingencies—that is, for unpredictable events—is crucial to facing the future. You cannot predict all the monkey wrenches that can foul up the gears. You should be prepared, as best you can, to make *interim alternative plans* that will still allow you to remain on your trajectory. Of course, you might ask, "How am I supposed to make alternative plans?

I can't predict the future." Well, you do what you can. Perhaps you put aside funds to tide you over in case you lose your college scholarship ("I'll get my grades back up next semester, and get that scholarship again"). Perhaps you apply to a Caribbean medical school, just in case you don't get into an American school ("One way or another, I'll be a doctor"). If a challenge suddenly arises that you couldn't have planned for, then you should be nimble enough to meet it—like the lawyer in the example above, you figure out a work-around.

Of course, sometimes your initial good choice can morph as you pursue it. While it's important not to give up when you encounter obstacles, it's also important to recognize that you won't be the same person at twenty-five or thirty—or at fifty or sixty—than you were at an earlier phase of your life. It's actually fun to reread your college application ("I'm going to be an anthropologist, and study Neanderthal teeth to see if they domesticated grains") and realize how your goals may have changed. The point is that you need to balance commitment and follow-through with an ability to *accept* change. You may be disappointed if your initial choice is no longer feasible, or if it just doesn't fit with your current self-conception. But then you should accept the change and make the most of new choices. So long as you don't frivolously change your mind, you will always have a shot at fulfillment. In fact, college is the place to explore *tentative* choices until you settle on some that work ("Anthropology doesn't do it for me, but I'm still fascinated by teeth, so I'm signing up for the pre-dental program"). Sometimes your choices will partially but not entirely shift ("Hey, teeth are still teeth, right?"). You're in a phase of self-discovery.

Yet no matter how your professional goals shift, fulfillment on an emotional level will always depend on having solid friendships and, probably, intimate relationships with people you love. In fact, as life seems to swirl around you, and change winks from behind every good choice that you *think* you've made, you should be able to find support in other people. Cultivate these people, even while you're pursuing unrelated plans for your future. This chapter talks about feeling fulfilled in many dimensions. These dimensions will shift in importance as you focus on one or another aspect of your life. Yet it's still important to find some rough balance among them. For example, the lawyer who was determined to make partner kept up with his friends. He also took on some pro bono work ("Okay, my clients are all Wall Street moguls, but I try to vindicate my values by helping out the less privileged"). We're all complex. Feeling fulfilled reflects that complexity.

What steps can you take toward making the most of your choices?—You're unlikely to feel fulfilled quickly—say, a day or a week or a month—after making a good choice. Probably your follow-through will continue for years until your mastery becomes apparent. That's the case with professional dancers and musicians, who practice continually even after they suddenly burst onto the stage and make it all seem effortless.

Here's an important principle: To make your performance *seem* effortless, you need to invest a huge amount of effort. Then you just *keep* working at it. Even the greatest dancers, like Nureyev and Baryshnikov, practiced for hours every single day to maintain their skill.

Practice is a type of learning. It's not rote, even though you may feel like you're doing the same thing again and again. Rather, it's intense focus. You narrow down exactly what you need to keep working on. Ice skaters and gymnasts practice (and practice and practice) their routines to get the tiniest nuance just right. Practice allows them to create muscle memory, so they can reproduce their moves without conscious thought. By creating muscle memory, they're creating a habit.

In his famous book, *Outliers: The Story of Success*, Malcolm Gladwell states: "Ten thousand hours is the magic number of greatness." He means that to be considered truly experienced in your field, you must have practiced for ten thousand hours. His examples include Bill Gates (who founded Microsoft and changed how we process information), and the Beatles (no explanation required). Of course, whether or not you take Gladwell literally, he makes a good point—success requires a *lot* of practice. That's not fake-it-till-you-make-it practice, but real, dedicated hard work and attention to detail. You're so involved that you virtually fuse with what you're practicing. Bill Gates was as much a computer geek as he was a guy from Seattle. In "Among School Children," the poet William Butler Yeats puts this idea succinctly when he asks, "How can we know the dancer from the dance?" suggesting that creative acts are so intimately connected with the actor that to separate the two is nearly impossible.

If you stop and think, this principle applies to all sorts of undertakings, even those that are not highly technical. For example, becoming someone's good friend takes work—what fun things can you do together? how can you best support them? It can take years to "learn" someone, and to develop the trust that makes friendship possible. This is even more so in an intimate relationship, where each partner relies on the other intensely (sometimes exclusively), and expects so much more.

Learning a foreign language is another example. You could buy an app and practice pronunciation. You could read French newspapers and watch French movies. You could start a French book club. There are so many ways to practice that you should never get bored. When you feel confident enough, go to lectures in French—for example, there are Alliance Française chapters all over the United States. You can also find them on several French YouTube channels.

The point is that if you want to succeed at anything that can be a source of fulfillment—from computers, to dancing, to friendship—you'll first have to put in the work. You'll have to practice, learn, revise, repeat, until you get it right. Then you'll have to keep practicing because there's no status quo when life (or business) keeps changing and you have to keep up.

Does all this sound tiring? Are you wondering, "Is it all worth it?" If it means enough to you, then it is worth it. But when it ceases to be sufficiently important to who you are—when the dancer and the dance finally come apart—you can switch gears and find another source of fulfillment. Take, for example, Bill Gates. When he finally had enough of running Microsoft, he formed what is now known as the Gates Foundation, with over $75 billion in assets. Once again, he set out to change the world, this time with a different focus—tackling intractable issues of public health. However, his experience at Microsoft was crucial, since had learned how to navigate international politics. He learned how to make stuff happen.

The great tennis stars Venus and Serena Willams are just as much larger than life. Together, they have won every championship that it's possible to win in their sport, and they have done so with infinite grace. Everyone loves them. But what's impressive is that even while they were gifted with immense natural talent, their abilities were honed through years of practice. As we learned from the biopic *King Richard*, they started as middle-class kids who—literally—never dropped the ball. They worked and worked until they were ready to burst onto the world stage. They remained on that stage as peak performers longer than almost any of their peers. When Serena had to withdraw from playing after a difficult pregnancy, she fought her way back. She kept her eyes on her goal of playing at the top of her game.

After her tennis career, Serena became a venture capitalist, investing in over sixty start-ups. Venus became an entrepreneur, nutritionist, and advocate for gender equality and mental health concerns. Having developed drive and ambition, they never stopped moving, even if they changed direction later in life. But you might ask, "Will they ever feel fulfilled?" Even they may be unable to tell you. But the point is that without their extraordinary journey and huge personal commitment of time, energy, and belief in themselves, they couldn't have done what they've done so far.

Of course, women like Venus and Serena Williams demonstrate that if we're restless and creative, enough may never be Enough. We'll always want more. We won't ever feel fulfilled—or, we will for a while . . . until some new goal emerges. For some people, fulfillment is not just experienced in many dimensions; it's a temporal, perhaps a lifelong process. But that's okay. These people thrive on buzz. They'd probably just say, "I can't help it if I see around corners. If that's where the future is, then I want part of it."

"Later" is never the right time—Most people aren't Venus or Serena Williams. Still, when something matters to you, it's not enough to say, "Well, that's on my to-do list." When you defer taking responsibility for your life (and so defer making the most of a good choice), you'll find that the "right" time to get busy keeps receding. Other choices intervene. Now is the right time. Pay attention. Be deliberate. No one suggests that you should shun fun, but you'll discover soon enough that life is too short *not* to make the most of your good choices.

The present and the future—*your* present and *your* future—are continuous. If you commit yourself today to following through on good choices, the consequences will be apparent as you mature. You will have accomplished something. Maybe not exactly what you set out to do (life has a way of throwing curve balls), but still something that can make your life more fulfilling. Of course, you caught that qualifier "more." Do you ever really feel fulfilled? If any case, does the feeling last? In *Towards Happiness—A Psychoanalytic Approach to Finding Your Way*, we argued that happiness comes and goes. It's affected by circumstances, and by your state of mind on any given day. But, as we also argued, this is why you should never give up. If it's finally time to change course, then now is the time to do it.

There's that old saw, "Today is the first day of the rest of your life." It's true. If your dreams haven't come true—or if they have and then they turned sour—dream again. That's easy to say. But what other choice do you have? Think of that other old cliché, "If you have lemons, make lemonade." Don't just stare at the lemons (which, admittedly, are not cultured pearls) and feel sorry for yourself. When you wallow in grief, people will offer emotional support, but they won't get excited about your new plans. They won't climb on board and offer useful, maybe even transformative advice. Feel free to linger in the five stages of grief (denial, anger, bargaining, depression, and acceptance) . . . and then bust out of them. Once you've accepted that your situation is your situation, it's time to move on. It's time to make new choices.

It's still a lot better than giving up. You don't want to waste the present. If you apply yourself, you may still create something wonderful. What's better than a great surprise?

Takeaways—Making the most of good choices can lead to a fulfilling life. You can maximize your choices by taking actions that help you accomplish what you set out to. This may involve years of practice. But if your goals matter to you, then the effort is worthwhile. If you finally discover that you can't meet your goals, or that you want to change them, then that's okay. Just pick up and start again. Don't give up.

Questions to ask yourself and to discuss:

- Have I made good choices, or am I undecided about what will make me feel fulfilled?

- How do I define fulfillment—succeeding in business, having great friends, being creative?
- If I've made good choices, am I committed to pursuing them?
- Do I practice enough, and try to accumulate useful experience?
- Am I prepared to define a whole new set of choices if my current choices don't work out for me?
- Do I have a support network to help me reach my goals?

Further reading

Daniels, Peter. *How to Reach Your Life Goals: Keys to Help You Fulfill Your Dreams.* Honor Books, 2023.

Friedberg, Ahron, MD, with Sandra Sherman. *Everyday Leadership: Taking Charge in the Real World.* Routledge, 2024.

Friedberg, Ahron, MD, with Sandra Sherman. *Towards Happiness—A Psychoanalytic Approach to Finding Your Way.* Routledge, 2022.

Gladwell, Malcolm. *Outliers: The Story of Success.* Little, Brown and Company, 2008.

King Richard. Directed by Reinaldo Marcus Green, 2021.

Novitskaya, Ilona. *Embracing an Effective Life: Reaching Your Goals While Staying True to Yourself.* Self published, 2025.

Conclusion

In this *Guide*, the word "now" appears on nearly every page. It's the pivot on which this *Guide* turns. It's a polite imperative.

But why all this insistence? What's so crucial about the present tense? Isn't life a long expanse filled with possibility?

It can be, provided you get a good start. You need to make possibility *possible,* even as demands on your time and capacities nudge you into predictable, tractable grooves.

"Now" embodies the idea that what you do as a young person—whether it's eating right or building a community—has a huge effect on the person you want to become. If you start now, when your brain is still developing and you're not boxed in by dead-end choices, you won't end up with a case of "If only I'd . . ." (the list of missed opportunities can be endless). Rather, you'll retain a sense of possibility, even as you emphasize *some* possibilities over others. Your perspective will remain optimistic. You'll maintain a robust sense of Now. The present will seem porous—as open to the future as it's necessarily been shaped by the past.

You won't feel stuck. You'll feel like you've built up strong personal characteristics so that you can face challenges and get past them. If you experience regret, you'll find a work-around and retain a forward-facing momentum. You'll be up for a new start—in a new Now—if that's what it takes to thrive.

You'll keep growing—not just because you may have to, but because at different times you may want to renew yourself and take a different path. If you start building your skills in that direction now, they'll be there when you need them. In *Eat, Pray, Love*, Elizabeth Gilbert goes on a journey of self-discovery, bursting out of her comfort zone to discover a resilience she never knew she had. But she had it. It made possible an entirely new life, based on off-the-charts experiences. It's a place you can be in too (maybe minus off-the-charts) if you start now.

Of course, this *Guide* suggests that there's a lot to work on. You can't do it all at once. But neither do you have to reinvent the wheel and struggle to keep up skills that you struggled to acquire. Another big-time word in this *Guide*, "habit" (and its variations), is used even more often, and is meant to suggest that if you make good choices now and turn them into routines, it will be progressively easier to become your best self. You'll learn to integrate an array of good qualities into a self that you enjoy inhabiting.

What does it mean to integrate your good qualities?— You should *integrate* your best qualities so that they reinforce each other and make sense together. This means approaching your life holistically (from a 360-degree perspective), so that empathy becomes a part of community building; eating right is an everyday component of how you avoid mood swings;

and developing core moral values leads naturally to finding healthy, sustaining relationships. At the highest level, a holistic approach involves your recognizing—and putting into practice—the mind/body connection that this *Guide* has focused on, one way or another, in virtually every chapter. Training yourself to avoid sugary processed foods ("I'll skip the Oreos and take the peach") is a great way to live in your body sensibly and treat it with care. After all, it's the only body you'll ever have. How you treat it now will affect how you live in it later.

The chapters in this *Guide* build on each other because we must integrate our good qualities (which we spent so much time developing) into an MO that defines who we are. We can't say, "I want a good relationship, but I'm not big on empathy," or "I've got good moral values, but they don't determine the communities I join." Saying such stuff just sounds weird. As you think about what you've read, think about how you make sense of each chapter in terms of the others.

For example, ask yourself: "Am I practicing empathy in my relationships?" "Am I learning *how* to build good habits, so they're there when I want to avoid mood swings?" "Do I practice self-reflection as part of making the right choices?" You know how, when you read a novel for the second time, disparate pieces fall into place? You think, "Oh, now I get it." The same is true here. The chapters are about themselves and, to a degree, about each other. Together, they reflect the holistic approach to life that's essential if you want to be a success.

Naturally, such an approach takes work. It requires that you not slack off ("I'll get back to empathy eventually—right now I'm focused on myself"). It requires that you take the long view, rather than opting for short-term advantages that can easily fizzle. You know that school takes work. Well, so does life.

Everyone is different—Each of us has our own genetic endowment. We have different degrees of material advantage. Our parents may be nurturing or . . . not. Perhaps we experienced trauma that left us with PTSD. We all start from different places. "Now" is different for everyone. But as this *Guide* tries to show, you can develop resiliency skills that will move the needle on your life. Starting where you are, you can be in a better place by reflecting on the place you're in now, then devising a way to bounce upward. In our book, *Through a Screen Darkly: Psychoanalytic Reflection During the Pandemic,* the final essay is called "Acceptance." It recounts how people hit hard by the pandemic accept where they are, then "bounce" in new directions. They show that resilience is not just bouncing back to where you were; it's also about finding somewhere else that's potentially advantageous. This *Guide* suggests that if you remain flexible and open to new options (think of Elizabeth Gilbert), you'll find some that work for you. You can keep possibility possible no matter your starting point.

Possibilities vs. choices—Of course, as we grow, our choices narrow the possibilities we can choose from. If we choose to be a doctor, for example, it's much harder to start over and go to law school (if for no other reason than we probably have a mountain of debt to pay off). As this *Guide* demonstrates, it's important to choose wisely. Chapter I examines the process of making good choices—choosing *is* a process, rather than some fast, instinctive response to what seems attractive. In a way, making good choices is a twist on the idea of "Now," since it requires that we take account of the needs of some future self that we haven't yet have grown into. It requires a kind of maturity that we don't yet have. Like living holistically, making good choices is work. We do the best that we can, based on all the options after we've weighed all the risks. But at the same time, it's important to remain flexible. Even if we feel committed to one choice over another, we should know how to change course if the choice turns out to be wrong.

There are many reasons why a choice may not be right in the long run. The market for your skills may change. You may finally just be bored. The point is not to feel guilty about change. You are in charge of your life. "But what about my responsibilities to my family? I can't just leave the practice of law and become an artist." That's hard. Yet, if you work out your concerns *together* with those toward whom you feel responsible, you may still find a better place. Maybe you can cut back on your legal practice. Maybe you can go to art school at night and *then* become a really good artist. Learning how to be your best self as circumstances change is an important skill. It's yet another version of resilience.

Be fully in the present—If you're caught up in the past ("I should have . . ."), you may become paralyzed by it ("I should have . . . so now I won't do anything—it'll just be second best"). You may just sit around and sulk. But while you should allow yourself to feel regret, and even guilt, you should finally just move on. Give yourself to the moment. Pursue the possibilities it presents. Even imagine possibilities that may not yet be clear. The point is to be engaged with what's happening around you. If a relationship doesn't work out, be open to other people. *Act* like you're open to them. They may become interested in you—at which point, make your best effort to discover if you'd like to become more involved. If nothing else, you may have a good time, which is itself a defense against old encroaching memories.

Set goals—This *Guide* talks a lot about setting realistic goals. Goals are necessarily forward-facing. They reflect who you want to be. They help you make the present—that is, Now—into a useful instrument for becoming who you want to be. They give meaning and orientation to what you do every day. In this sense, goals are a bridge between now and the future, and make you feel like you're growing.

Of course, goals can pitch into reverse and become a source of disappointment. It happens. But so does resilience, provided you've cultivated it. We keep coming back to resilience since it's so important to maintaining the sound mind component of the sound mind/sound body equation. Don't be afraid to set lofty (albeit realistic) goals. Just develop the capacity to recover your momentum if you fail. Disappointment is not your enemy; remaining stuck is. You can learn from your mistakes.

Health and wellness is a balance—This *Guide* talks about balance:

- A diet that suits your body type and activity level—an Oreo a day is okay, but don't overdo it
- Your being open and engaged with others, even as you make time for self-reflection
- Being empathetic, while making sure to look after yourself

- Making choices, where you should balance risks and rewards

At every turn, striking a balance is key. The point is not to live at the edge, which can be exciting but dangerous. Rather, it's to live well, somewhere in the middle where you can thrive within the limits of your personal resources. Should you try to stretch those limits? Of course, but not recklessly. You learn as you go along, striking new balances as you become more sure-footed.

Ultimately, health and wellness require paying attention, so that when the balance seems off you can adjust it. After a while, you develop an intuition about yourself ("I just know I have to fix things"), and you know when things are beyond your control and you should reach out to someone who can help. It's okay to display vulnerability. Health and wellness are never static, and being open about yourself is the first step to a new, better you.

Returning to Now—This conclusion started by suggesting that Now can make a difference to the rest of your life. It further suggested, somewhat more radically, that making good choices now will fuse the present with a still uncertain future, making it more plausible and tractable once you finally get there. Think about that connection. Try to make the most of it. This *Guide* suggests ways to do that. You can make each suggestion your own, based on your sense of self. Part of becoming who you want to be—part of feeling fulfilled—is finding an MO that suits you, that you can turn into routines that work for you. If you work at what works for you, you'll be off to a great start.

Index

Notes

....
....
....
....
....
....
....
....
....
....
....
....
....
....
....
....
....
....
....
....
....
....

Notes

Notes

....
....
....
....
....
....
....
....
....
....
....
....
....
....
....
....
....
....
....
....
....

Notes

Notes

....

....

....

....

....

....

....

....

....

....

....

....

....

....

....

....

....

....

....

Notes

Notes

....
....
....
....
....
....
....
....
....
....
....
....
....
....
....
....
....
....
....
....
....
....
....